WISDOM FOR LIFE

WISDOM
FOR LIFE

Editorial Selection by
Lynnette Evans

**CHARTWELL
BOOKS, INC.**

Published by
CHARTWELL BOOKS, INC.
A Division of **BOOK SALES, INC.**
114 Northfield Avenue, Edison, New Jersey 08837

ISBN 0-7858-1812-X

Text copyright © CRW Publishing Limited 2004

Editorial selection by Lynnette Evans
Typeset in Great Britain by Antony Gray
Printed and bound in China

Contents

I want to be a rock, dislodged from the highest part of the woods. I want to crash and tumble my disregarding way through the trees, bumping and bouncing and yelling out my journey, calling out to the river of my imminent surging, splashing, crashing arrival. And the river and I are one, yet apart, waterfalling together.

LYNNETTE EVANS

Living Wisely

All Nature is but Art, unknown to thee;
All chance, direction, which thou canst not see;
All discord, harmony not understood;
All partial evil, universal good;
And, spite of pride, in erring reason's spite,
One truth is clear, WHATEVER IS, IS RIGHT.

Alexander Pope (1688–1744)

We learn wisdom from failure, much more than
from success; we often discover what will do, by
finding out what will not do, and probably he who
never made a mistake never made a discovery.

Samuel Smiles (1812–1904)

Does the Eagle know what is in the pit?
Or wilt thou go ask the Mole:
Can Wisdom be put in a silver rod?
Or Love in a golden bowl?

William Blake (1757–1827)

Take the good until you find something better, and in search for something better do not let the good slip away from you or die out. If you disregard it despite its worth, and pursue something better, what you had escapes you; but if you remain attached to what is good, you will always have it if nothing better follows.

Paracelsus (1493–1541)

Every now and then go away, have a little relaxation, for when you come back to your work, your judgement will be surer, since to remain constantly at your work will cause you to lose power and judgement.

Leonardo da Vinci (1452–1519)

Sow good, even on an unworthy soil; for it will
    not be fruitless wherever it is sown.
Verily, good, though it remain long buried, none
    will reap but he who sowed it.

The Thousand and One Nights

Keep to truth, although it scorch thee
with the fire of threatening;

The Assemblies of Al Hariri

What is the price of Experience do men buy
  it for a song
Or wisdom for a dance in the street? No it
  is bought with the price
Of all that a man hath, his house his wife
  his children
Wisdom is sold in the desolate market
  where none come to buy
And in the wither'd field where the farmer
  ploughs for bread in vain

William Blake (1757–1827)

He who binds to himself a joy
Does the winged life destroy
But he who kisses the joy as it flies
Lives in eternity's sun rise

William Blake (1757–1827)

Not everything is good because it is old,
Nor poems always bad by being new.
Good men try both before they make their choice,
While the fool but takes the view of others.

Sanskrit poem (author unknown)

It is easy in the world to follow the world's opinions; it is easy in solitude to follow our own; but the great man is he who in the midst of the crowd keeps with perfect sweetness the independence of solitude.

Ralph Waldo Emerson (1803–82)

Hide the good you do, and make known
the good done to you.

Author unknown

Flee with thy life if thou fearest oppression,
  and leave the house to tell its builder's fate.
Thou wilt find, for the land that that thou
  quittest, another;
But no soul wilt thou find to replace thine own.

The Thousand and One Nights

There is but one cause of human failure, and
that is man's lack of faith in his true self.

William James (1842–1910)

Study depends on the goodwill of the student, a quality that cannot be secured by compulsion.

Quintilian (35–100)

Seek knowledge, for learning is a good deed before God; to disclose it is praise, to seek it is worship, to teach it is charity.

Author unknown

Violence is infamous; its result is ever uncertain, and no-one can act justly when actuated by hatred.

Antar: A Bedouin Romance

We are what we think. All that we are arises with our thoughts. With our thoughts we make the world. Speak or act with a pure mind and happiness will follow you as your shadow, unshakeable.

The Dhammapada

Risk! Risk anything! Care no more for the opinions of others, for those voices. Do the hardest thing on earth for you. Act for yourself.

Katherine Mansfield (1888–1923)

Both in a good and a bad sense, the English are farther from a state of nature than any other modern people. They are, more than any other people, a product of civilization and discipline. England is the country in which social discipline has most succeeded, not so much in conquering, as in suppressing, whatever is liable to conflict with it. The English, more than any other people, not only act but feel according to rule.

John Stuart Mill (1806–73)

Where men of judgement creep and feel their way,
The positive pronounce without dismay.

William Cowper (1731–1800)

There is no writer that shall not perish, but what
his hand hath written endureth ever.
Write, therefore, nothing but what wilt please thee
when thou shall see it on the day of resurrection.

The Thousand and One Nights

Words are like leaves, and where they most
    abound,
Much fruit of sense beneath is rarely found.

Alexander Pope (1688–1744)

You are oblig'd to your imagination for more
    than three-fourths of your importance.

David Garrick (1717–79)

For there is no grace in a benefit
    that sticks to the fingers.

Lucius Seneca (*c.*4BC–AD65)

Scatter your favours on a fop,
Ingratitude's the certain crop.

Alexander Pope (1688–1744)

Knowledge and Wisdom, far from being one,
Have oft-times no connection. Knowledge dwells
In heads replete with thoughts of other men;
Wisdom in minds attentive to their own.

William Cowper (1731–1800)

Go to the ant, thou sluggard;
consider her ways, and be wise.

The Bible, Proverbs 6

A man I knew who lived upon a smile;
And well it fed him: he look'd plump and fair,
While rankest venom foam'd through every vein.

Edward Young (1683–1765)

The talkative listen to no one, for they are ever
speaking. And the first evil that attends those who
know not to be silent is, that they hear nothing.

Plutarch (c.46–120)

I have no spur
To prick the sides of my intent, but only
Vaulting ambition, which o'erleaps itself,
And falls on the other.

William Shakespeare (1564–1616)

And like the ocean, day by day receiving
Floods from all lands, which never overflows;
Its boundary line not leaping, and not leaving,
Fed by the rivers, but unswelled by those:
So is the perfect one.

Bhagavad Gita, Book 2

Man, proud man!
Dressed in a little brief authority:
Most ignorant of what he's most assured.
His glassy essence – Like an angry ape
Plays such fantastic tricks before high heaven
As make the angels weep.

William Shakespeare (1564–1616)

You cannot eat your cake and have it.

Plautus (c.250–184BC)

He that attends to his interior self,
That has a heart, and keeps it; has a mind
That hungers, and supplies it; and who seeks
A social, not dissipated life,
Has business.

William Cowper (1731–1800)

Every man has a bag hanging before him, in which
he puts his neighbour's faults, and another behind
him in which he stows his own.

William Shakespeare (1564–1616)

If I am right, Thy grace impart
Still in the right to stay:
If I am wrong, oh teach my heart
To find that better way.

Alexander Pope (1688–1744)

Great things are done when men and
   mountains meet;
This is not done by jostling in the street.

William Blake (1757–1827)

From these remarks it will be seen how greatly I differ, at once from those, who seeing the institutions of our ancestors to be bad for us, imagine that they were bad for those for whom they were made.

John Stuart Mill (1806–73)

When abasement is a thing not to be avoided, meet
    with it by asking of the great.
Thine honouring the great is no abasement of
    thyself; it is only abasement to honour the
    unworthy.

The Thousand and One Nights

When we mean to build,
We first survey the plot, then draw the model;
And when we see the figure of the house,
Then must we rate the cost of the erection:
Which if we find outweighs ability,
What do we then, but draw anew the model
In fewer offices; or at least, desist
To build at all?

William Shakespeare (1564–1616)

The wisest men in every age generally surpass in wisdom the wisest of any preceding age, because the wisest men possess and profit by the constantly increasing accumulation of the ideas of all ages . . .

John Stuart Mill (1806–73)

But Ignorance, begot
Of Darkness, blinding mortal men, binds down
Their souls to stupor, sloth and drowsiness.

Bhagavad Gita, Book 14

Ask yourself whether you are happy
and you cease to be so.

Author Unknown

Who, dwelling quiet eyed,
Stainless, serene, well-balanced, unperplexed,
Working with Me, yet from all works detached,
That man I love!

Bhagavad Gita, Book 12

My shrinking flesh complains
And murmurs to content so long;
My mind superior is to pains;
When I am weak, then am I strong.

Zilpha Elaw (c.1790–1847)

May those, whose holy task it is,
To guide impulsive youth,
Fail not to cherish in their souls
A reverence for truth;
For teachings which the lips impart
Must have their source within the heart.

Charlotte Forten (1837–1914)

True wisdom, which is never found at variance with rectitude, is as useful to women as to men; because it is necessary to the highest degree of happiness, which can never exist with ignorance.

Catherine Macaulay (1731–91)

Besides viewing the subject from a solely artistic point of view, a good writer of fiction must have lived an active and sympathetic life if she wishes her books to have strength and vitality in them.

Elizabeth Gaskell (1810–65)

There have been too many theories and thus we have become divided, which means the burial of all truth and all power.

George Sand (1804–76)

Even weak men when united are powerful.

Johann Schiller (1759–1805)

Dirt is not dirt, but only something in
the wrong place.

Henry John Temple
(1784–1865)

Don't be a cynic and disconsolate preacher.
Don't bewail and moan. Omit the negative
propositions. Nerve us with incessant
affirmatives. Don't waste yourself in
rejection, nor bark against the bad, but
chant the beauty of the good.

Ralph Waldo Emerson (1803–82)

Endeavour not to settle too many habits at once, lest by variety you confound them, and so perfect none.

John Locke (1632–1704)

Eyes will not see when the heart wishes them to be blind; desire conceals truth as darkness does the earth.

Lucius Seneca (c.4BC–AD65)

Faces are as legible as books, only they are read in much less time, and are much less likely to deceive us.

Johann Lavater (1741–1801)

That which can be done with perfect convenience and without loss, is not always the thing that most needs to be done, or which we are most imperatively required to do.

John Ruskin (1819–1900)

Superior powers of mind and profound study are of no use if they do not sometimes lead a person to different conclusions from those which are formed by ordinary powers of mind without study.

John Stuart Mill (1806–73)

Those people who are always improving never become great. Greatness is an eminence, the ascent to which is steep and lofty, and which a man must seize on at once by natural boldness and vigour, and not by patient, wary steps.

William Hazlitt (1778–1830)

Let your speech be always with grace, seasoned with salt, that ye may know how to answer every man.

The Bible, St Paul

It is with narrow-soul'd people as with narrow neck'd bottles; the less they have in them, the more noise they make in pouring it out.

Jonathan Swift (1667–1745)

It is with words as with sunbeams; the more they are condensed, the deeper they burn.

Robert Southey (1774–1843)

We are taxed twice as much by our idleness, three times as much by our pride, and four times as much by our folly: and from these taxes the Commissioners cannot ease or deliver us by allowing an abatement.

Benjamin Franklin (1706–90)

Revenge is a kind of wild justice.

Francis Bacon (1561–1626)

We are seldom sure that we sincerely meant
what we omitted to do.

Samuel Johnson (1709–84)

We are not to be astonished that the wise walk
more slowly in their road to virtue than fools in
their passage to vice; since passion drags us along,
while wisdom only points out the way.

Confucius (*c.* 551–748 BC)

We are not sent into this world to do anything into which we cannot put our hearts. We have certain work to do for our bread, and that is to be done strenuously; other work to do for our delight, and that is to be done heartily; neither is to be done by halves or shifts, but with a will; and what is not worth this effort is not be done at all.

John Ruskin (1819–1900)

Education is an admirable thing, but it is well to remember from time to time that nothing that is worth knowing can be taught.

Oscar Wilde (1854–1900)

There is nothing so ridiculous that has not at some time been said by some philosopher.

Oliver Goldsmith (1728–74)

We cannot prevent the black birds of evil from flying over our heads, but we can prevent them from building their nests in our hair.

Chinese Proverb

Dost thou think because thou art virtuous, there shall be no more cakes and ale?

William Shakespeare (1564–1616)

Verily never will Allah change the condition of a people until they change it themselves (with their own souls).

The Qu'ran 13:11

He who knows the light, and at the same time keeps the shade, will be the whole world's model.

Lao Tsze (*c*.604–531BC)

Whoso thus knows himself, and knows his soul,
Working through the qualities with Nature's
modes, the light hath come for him!
Whatever flesh he bears, never again
Shall he take on its load.

Bhagavad Gita, Book 13

He granteth wisdom to whom He pleaseth; and he
to whom wisdom is granted receiveth indeed a
benefit overflowing; but none will grasp the
message of understanding.

The Qu'ran 2:269

A book that is shut is but a block.

Proverb

Wine is a mocker, strong drink is raging: and
whosoever is deceived thereby is not wise.

The Bible, Proverbs 20:1

Miserable, to my mind, is the one who has
nowhere in his home where he can be alone,
where his mind can especially be; where he
can hide himself.

Michel de Montaigne (1533–92)

Happy is the man that findeth wisdom, and the man that getteth understanding. For the merchandise of it is better than the merchandise of silver, and the gain thereof than fine gold. She is more precious than rubies: and all the things thou canst desire are not to be compared unto her.

The Bible, Proverbs 3:13–15

When in the world goodness is recognized to be good, straightway there is evil. And thus, in like manner, existence and non-existence mutually originate each other; so also difficulty and ease, long and short, high and low, treble and bass, before and after.

Lao Tsze (c.604–531 BC)

He who knows others is wise. He who knows himself is enlightened.

Lao Tsze (c.604–531BC)

If a man will begin with certainties, he shall end in doubts; but if he will be content to begin with doubts, he shall end in certainties.

Francis Bacon (1561–1626)

The man who never alters his opinion is like standing water, and breeds reptiles of the mind.

William Blake (1757–1827)

How do you like this cold weather? I hope you have all been earnestly praying for it as a salutary relief from the dreadfully mild and unhealthy season preceding it . . . and that now you will all draw into the fire, complain in that you never felt such bitterness of cold before . . . and wish the mild weather back again with all your hearts.

Jane Austen (1776–1817)

I am happiest when I am idle. I could live for months without performing any kind of labour, and at the expiration of that time I should feel fresh and vigorous enough to go right on in the same way for numerous more months.

Charles Farrer Browne (1836–68)

When a man's busy, why, leisure
Strikes him as wonderful pleasure;
'Faith, and at leisure once is he?
Straightway he wants to be busy.

Robert Browning (1812–89)

And obey Allah and His Messenger; and fall
into no disputes, lest ye lose heart and your
power depart; and be patient and
persevering: for Allah is with those who
patiently persevere:

The Qu'ran 8:46

No one can be perfectly free till all are free; no one can be perfectly moral till all are moral; no one can be perfectly happy till all are happy.

Herbert Spencer (1820–1903)

For God's sake give me the young man who has enough brains to make a fool of himself!

Robert Louis Stevenson (1850–94)

Woe unto you, scribe and Pharisees, hypocrites! For ye make clean the outside of the cup and of the platter, but within they are full of extortion and excess. Thou blind Pharisee, cleanse first that which is within the cup and platter, that the outside of them may be clean also.

The Bible, Jesus, Matthew 23:25–26

He who acts
Free from self-seeking, humble, resolute,
Steadfast, in good or evil hap the same,
Content to do aright – he 'truly' acts.

Bhagavad Gita, Book 18

It makes a tremendous emotional and practical difference to one whether one accept the universe in the drab discoloured way of stoic resignation to necessity, or with the passionate happiness of Christian saints.

William James (1842–1910)

And so accept everything which happens, even if it seems disagreeable, because it leads to this, the health of the universe and to the prosperity and felicity of Zeus. For he would not have brought on any man what he has brought, if it were not useful for the whole.

Marcus Aurelius (121–180)

Truth is within ourselves; it takes no rise
From outward things, whate'er you may believe,
There is an inmost centre in us all,
Where truth abides in fullness.

Robert Browning (1812–89)

What renders me liable to great disaster is my
person; so that if I had no person (body, personal
importance), what disaster could I have?

Lao Tsze (c.604–531BC)

Where men are enlightened with the true light, they renounce all desire and choice, and commit and commend themselves and all things to the eternal Goodness . . . Such men are in a state of freedom, because they have lost the fear of pain or hell, and the hope of reward in heaven, and are living . . . in the perfect freedom of fervent love.

Theologica Germanica (Sixteenth century)

He who sees
How action may be rest, rest action – he
Is wisest mid his kind: he hath the truth!

Bhagavad Gita, Book 4

As near as I can get at it, to be a reasonable being is to laugh when your heart aches; it is to give confidence and receive none; it is faithfully to keep your own promises and never mind such a trifle as having promises broken to you. It is never to have or to promulgate a dissenting opinion. It is either to be born a fool, or in lack of that to become a hypocrite, trying to become a 'reasonable being'.

Sarah Parton (1811–72)

The only perfect life is that of inner wisdom, which makes one thing as indifferent to us as another, and thus leads to rest, to peace, and to Nirvana.

Buddha (*c.*563–483BC)

It had begun to be recognised, with a great burst of enthusiasm and astonishment, that, after all, Mill and Herbert Spencer had not said the last word on all things in heaven and earth.

Mary Ward (1851–1920)

Having Enough

Let us all be happy, and live within our means, even if we have to borrow the money to do it with.

Charles Farrer Browne (1836–68)

You never know what is enough unless you know what is more than enough.

William Blake (1757–1827)

Happiness resides not in possessions and not in gold, the feeling of happiness dwells in the soul.

Democritus (*c.*470–400BC)

When my wealth faileth, no friend assisteth me;
     but when it aboundeth, all men are my friends.
How many enemies for the sake of wealth have
     consorted with me!
And my companion, in the time of want, hath
     abandoned me!

The Thousand and One Nights

Woe to every (kind of) scandalmonger and
     backbiter,
Who pileth up wealth and layeth it by,
Thinking that his wealth would make him last
     for ever!
By no means! He will be sure to be thrown
     into that which Breaks to Pieces.

The Qu'ran 104:1–4

And he gave it for his opinion, that whoever could make two ears of corn, or two blades of grass to grow upon a spot of ground where only one grew before, would deserve better of mankind and do more essential service to his country, than the whole race of politicians put together.

Jonathan Swift (1667–1745)

When Fortune is liberal to thee, be thou liberal to
    all others before she escape from thee;
For liberality will not annihilate thy wealth when
    she is favourable; nor avarice preserve it when
    she deserteth thee.

The Thousand and One Nights

Generosity . . . adorns; but meanness . . . dishonours; the noble rewards, but the base disappoints; the princely entertains, but the niggard frights away; the liberal nourishes, but the churl pains; giving relieves, but deferring torments; blessing protects, and praise purifies; the honourable repays, for repudiation abases; the rejection of him who should be respected is error; a denial to the sons of hope is outrage; and none is miserly but the fool, and none is foolish but the miser; and none hoards but the wretched; for the pious clenches not his palms.

The Assemblies of Al–Hariri

A fine and slender net the spider weave,
Which little and light animals receives;
And if she catch a common bee or fly
They with a piteous groan and murmur die;
But if a wasp or hornet she entrap,
They tear her cords like Sampson and escape;
So, like a fly, the poor offender dies,
But, like the wasp, the rich escapes and flies.

Sir John Denham (1615–69)

The Sacrifice
Which Knowledge pays is better than great gifts
Offered by wealth, since gift's worth, o my Prince,
Lies in the mind which gives, the will that serves.

Bhagavad Gita, Book 4

Not tonight – I have very poor and unhappy brains for drinking: I could well wish courtesy would invent some other custom of entertainment. I have drunk but one cup tonight, and – behold what innovation it makes here: I am unfortunate in the infirmity, and are not to task my weakness with any more.

William Shakespeare (1564–1616)

Judges and senates have been bought for gold;
Esteem and love were never to be sold.

Alexander Pope (1688–1744)

Let a man who wants to find abundance of employment, procure a woman and a ship; for no two things do produce more trouble if you begin to equip them; neither are these two things ever equipped enough, nor is the largest amount of equipment sufficient for them.

Plautus (*c*.250–184BC)

Poor and content, is rich, and rich enough;
But riches, fineless, is as poor as winter,
To him that ever fears he shall be poor.

William Shakespeare (1564–1616)

The joys springing from sense-life are but
    quickening wombs
Which breed sure griefs: those joys begin and
    end.

Bhagavad Gita, Book 5

My father when our fortune smiled,
With jewels deck'd his eyeless child;
Their glittering worth the world might see,
But ah, they had no charms for me;
A trickling tear bedew'd my arm;
I felt it, and my heart was warm.
And sure the gem to me most dear,
Was a kind father's pitying tear.

John Collet (c.1725–80)

If thou ask a favour, ask it of the generous, who
   hath known, unceasingly, riches and opulence;
For asking of the generous is productive of
   honour, and asking of the base is productive
   of disgrace.

The Thousand and One Nights

Books, dear books,
Have been, and are my comforts; morn and night,
Adversity, prosperity, at home,
Abroad, health, sickness, good or ill report,
The same firm friends, the same refreshment rich,
And source of consolation

Pliny (Junior) (62–113)

Which of you, intending to build a tower, sitteth
  not down first and counteth the cost, whether
  he have sufficient to finish it?
Lest haply, after he hath laid the foundation, and is
  not able to finish it, all that behold it begin to
  mock him, saying, this man began to build, and
  was not able to finish.

The Bible, Luke 14:28-30

Dress drains our cellar dry
And keeps our larder lean; puts out our fires,
And introduces hunger, frost and woe,
Where peace and hospitality might reign.

William Cowper (1731–1800)

Nothing is thought rare
Which is not new and followed; yet we know
That what was worn some twenty years ago
Comes into grace again.

Francis Beaumont (1584–1616) &
John Fletcher (1579–1625)

For want of a nail, the shoe was lost;
For want of the shoe, the horse was lost;
For want of the horse, the rider was lost,
For want of the rider, the battle was lost;
For want of the battle, the kingdom was lost;
And all from the want of a horseshoe nail.

Author Unknown

It is a familiar fact, that the vulgar, in all parts of the world . . . do as their betters do . . . think as their betters think: and this very word 'betters', is speaking proof of the fact which we allege – meaning, as it does, not their 'wisers', or their 'honesters' but their 'richers' and those placed in authority over them.

John Stuart Mill (1806–73)

Only with him, Great Prince,
Whose senses are not swayed by things of sense;
Only with him who holds his mastery,
Shows wisdom perfect.

Bhagavad Gita, Book 2

From the earliest periods of the nations of modern Europe, all worldly power has belonged to one particular class, the wealthy class.

John Stuart Mill (1806–73)

If one ponders on objects of the sense, there
    springs
Attraction; from attraction grows desire
Desire flames to fierce passion, passion breeds
Recklessness; then the memory, all betrayed,
Lets noble purpose go, and saps the mind,
Till purpose, mind, and man are all undone.

Bhagavad Gita, Book 2

The unvowed, the passion-bound,
Seeking a fruit from works, are fastened down.

Bhagavad Gita, Book 5

For although mankind, in all ages except those of transition, are ever ready to obey and love those whom they recognize as better able to govern them, than they are to govern themselves, it is not in human nature to yield a willing obedience to men whom you think no wiser than yourself . . .

John Stuart Mill (1806–73)

The elements, the conscious life, the mind, the
    unseen vital force, the nine strange gates of the
    body, and the five domains of sense;
Desire, dislike, pleasure and pain, and thought
    deep-woven, and persistency of being;
These all are wrought on Matter by the Soul!

Bhagavad Gita, Book 13

I confess I sometimes wish for a little conversation;
but I reflect that the commerce of the world gives
more uneasiness than pleasure.

Lady Mary Wortley Montagu (1689–1762)

Economy no more means saving money than it means spending money. It means the administration of a house, its stewardship; spending or saving, that is, whether money or time, or anything else, to the best possible advantage.

John Ruskin (1819–1900)

Fame, we may understand, is no sure test of merit, but only a probability of such: it is an accident, not a property, of a man: like light, it can give little or nothing, but at most may show what is given; often it is but a false glare, dazzling the eyes of the vulgar, lending, by casual extrinsic splendour, the brightness and manifold glance of the diamond to pebbles of no value.

Thomas Carlyle (1795–1881)

Steadfastly the will
Must toil thereto, till efforts end in ease,
And thought has passed from thinking. Shaking off
All longings bred by dreams of fame and gain,
Shutting the doorways of the senses close
With watchful ward; so, step by step, it comes
To gift of peace assured.

Bhagavad Gita, Book 6

Fortune turns like a mill-wheel, and he that was
yesterday at the top lies today at the bottom.

Spanish Proverb

The tendency of the human to the worship of power, is well understood. It is a matter of common complaint, that even the Supreme Being is adored by an immense majority as the Almighty, not as the All-good . . .

John Stuart Mill (1806–73)

Power often deprives a man of all spirit and virtue. It is hard for an empty bag to stand upright.

Benjamin Franklin (1706–90)

The civilised nation consists broadly of mob, money-collecting machine, and capitalist; and when the mob wishes to spend money for any purpose, it sets its money-collecting machine to borrow the money it needs from the capitalist, who lends it on condition of taxing the mob generation after generation.

John Ruskin (1819–1900)

Ensnared in nooses of a hundred idle hopes,
Slaves to their passion and their wrath, they buy
Wealth with base deeds, to glut hot appetites.
'Thus much, today' they say, 'we gained!'
. . . So they speak . . . and so they fall.

Bhagavad Gita, Book 16

That we should find our national existence depend on selling manufactured cotton a farthing an ell cheaper than any other people, is a most narrow stand for a great nation to base itself on.

Thomas Carlyle (1795–1881)

Going by railroad I do not consider as travelling at all; it is merely 'being sent' to a place, and very little from becoming a parcel.

John Ruskin (1819–1900)

Gold, like the sun, which melts wax and hardens clay, expands great souls and contracts bad hearts.

Antoine de Rivarol (1753–1801)

Liberty is of more value than any gifts;
and to receive gifts is to lose it.

Muslih Addin Saadi (*c.*1184–1292)

Prayer that craves a particular commodity, anything less than all god, is vicious. As a means to effect a private end, it is meanness and theft.

Ralph Waldo Emerson (1803–82)

A cynical, mercenary, demagogic, corrupt press will produce in time a people as base as itself.

Joseph Pulitzer (1847–1911)

Rent is that portion of the earth, which is paid to the landlord for the use of the original and indestructible powers of the soil.

David Ricardo (1772–1823)

Jesus said unto him, If thou wilt be perfect, go and sell that thou hast, and give to the poor, and thou shalt have treasure in heaven: and come and follow me. But when the young man heart that saying, he went away sorrowful: for he had great possessions.

The Bible, Jesus, Matthew 19:21–22

. . . a mind that letteth go what others prize;
And equanimity, and charity
Which spieth no man's faults; and tenderness
Towards all that suffer: a contented heart,
Fluttered by no desires; a bearing mild,
Modest, and grave, with manhood nobly mixed,
With patience, fortitude and purity;
An unrevengeful spirit, never given to rate itself
   too high;
Such be the signs . . . of him whose feet are set
On that fair path which leads to heavenly birth.

Bhagavad Gita, Book 16

Poverty consists in feeling poor.

Ralph Waldo Emerson (1803–82)

We need examples of people who, leaving Heaven to decide whether they are to rise in the world, decide for themselves that they will be happy in it, and have resolved to seek not greater wealth but simpler pleasure, not higher future but deeper felicity – to make the first of possessions self possession.

John Ruskin (1819–1900)

A king does not win because of his powerful army: a soldier does not triumph because of his strength.

The Bible, Psalm 33

Moses prayed: 'Our Lord! Thou has indeed bestowed on Pharaoh and his Chiefs splendour and wealth in the life of the Present, and so, our Lord, they mislead (men) from Thy Path. Deface, our Lord, the features of their wealth, and send hardness to their heats, so they will not believe until they see the grievous penalty'.

The Qu'ran 10:88

There are three distinguishable sources of moral influence – eminent wisdom and virtue, real or supposed; the power of addressing mankind in the name of religion; and finally, worldly power.

John Stuart Mill (1806–73)

Lay not up for yourselves treasures upon earth,
where moth and rust doth corrupt, and where
thieves break through and steal:
But lay up for yourselves treasures in heaven,
where neither moth nor rust doth corrupt, and
where thieves do not break through and steal:
For where your treasure is, there will your heart be
also.

The Bible, Jesus, Matthew 6:19–21

He who conquers others is strong. He who
conquers himself is mighty.
He who knows when he has enough is rich.

Lao Tsze (c.604–531BC)

Who is strong? He who subdues his passion. Who is rich? He who is satisfied with his lot.

The Talmud

Princes and kings, were it not for some source of dignity and highness, would be in danger of an ignominious fall. And here, one sees how nobility is rooted in (and entirely dependent upon) what is ignoble; and highness is founded and supported upon what is low.

Lao Tsze (c.604–531BC)

Be not pennywise; riches have wings, and sometimes they fly away of themselves, sometimes they must be set flying to bring in more.

Francis Bacon (1561–1626)

He may love riches that wanteth them, as much as he that hath them.

Richard Baxter (1615–91)

When gold and gems fill the hall none
can protect them.

Lao Tsze (c.604–531BC)

Power, like a desolating pestilence,
Pollutes what'er it touches; and obedience,
Bare of all genius, virtue, freedom, truth,
Makes slaves of men, and, of the human frame,
A mechanised automaton.

Percy Bysshe Shelley (1792–1822)

Like imperfect sleep which, instead of giving more strength to the head, doth but leave it the more exhausted, the result of mere operations of the imagination is but to weaken the soul.

St Theresa of Avila (1512–82)

Little by little, Tolstoy came to the settled conviction . . . that his trouble had not been with life in general, not with the common life of common men, but with the life of the upper, intellectual, artistic classes, the life which he had personally always led, the cerebral life, the life of conventionality, artificiality, and personal ambition.

William James (1842–1910)

I gave up the life of the conventional world, recognizing it to be no life, but a parody on life, which its superfluities simply keep us from comprehending.

Leo Tolstoy (1828–1910)

Woe unto you, scribes and Pharisees, hypocrites! For ye pay tithe of mint and anise and cummin, and have omitted the weightier matters of the law, judgement, mercy, and faith: these ought you to have done, and not to leave the other undone.

The Bible, Jesus, Matthew 23:23

Those who spend (freely), whether in prosperity, or in adversity; who restrain anger, and pardon (all) men; for Allah loves those who do good;

The Qu'ran 3:134

No race can prosper till it learns that there is as much dignity in tilling a field as in writing a poem.

Booker T. Washington (1856–1915)

Let no one use anything as if it were his private possession.

St Ignatius Loyola (1491–1556)

A man there was, though some did count him mad,
The more he gave away the more he had.

John Bunyan (1628–88)

The Future, the Past, and the Here and Now

Time is the most undefinable yet paradoxical of things: the past is gone, the future is not come, and the present becomes the past, even while we attempt to define it, and like the flash of the lightning, at once exists and expires.

Charles Colton (*c.*1780–1832)

What we are today comes from our thoughts of yesterday, and our present thoughts build our life of tomorrow. Our life is the creation of our mind.

Buddha (*c.*563–483BC)

To everything there is a season, and a time to
every purpose under the heaven:
A time to be born, and a time to die; a time to
plant, and a time to pluck up that which is
planted:
A time to kill, and a time to heal; a time to break
down, and a time to build up;
A time to weep, and a time to laugh; a time to
mourn, and a time to dance;
A time to cast away stones, and a time to gather
stones together; a time to embrace, and a time
to refrain from embracing;
A time to get, and a time to lose; a time to keep,
and a time to cast away;
A time to rend, and a time to sew; a time to keep
silence, and a time to speak;
A time to love, and a time to hate; a time of war,
and a time of peace.

The Bible, Ecclesiastes 3:1–8

Learn to be silence. Let your quiet
mind listen and absorb.

Pythagoras (*c*.582–500BC)

To dream of the person you would like to
be is to waste the person you are.

Author unknown

Confine yourself to the present.

Marcus Aurelius (121–180)

There is a Moment in each Day that Satan
    cannot find
Nor can his Watch Fiends find it, but the
    Industrious find
This Moment and it multiply.

William Blake (1757–1827)

To choose time is to save time.

Francis Bacon (1561–1626)

Ring out wild bells to the wild sky,
The flying cloud, the frosty light;
The year is dying in the night;
Ring out wild bells and let him die.

Ring out the old, ring in the new,
Ring happy bells across the snow;
The year is going, let him go;
Ring out the false, ring in the true.

Alfred, Lord Tennyson (1809–92)

Beware of desperate steps. The darkest day.
Live till tomorrow, will have pass'd away.

William Cowper (1731–1800)

The weary sun hath made a golden set,
And, by the bright track of his fiery car,
Gives token of a goodly day tomorrow.

William Shakespeare (1564–1616)

He thought on the days that were long since by,
When his limbs were strong, and his courage high.

Sir Walter Scott (1771–1832)

Redeem the misspent time that's past,
And live this day as 'twere thy last.

Author unknown

Look to this day, for it is life, the very life of
    life
In its brief course lie all the realities of
    existence
The joy of growth
The splendour of action
The glory of power
For yesterday is but a memory
And tomorrow is only a vision
But today well lived makes every yesterday a
    memory of happiness
And every tomorrow a vision of hope.
Look well, therefore, to this day.

Sanskrit poem (Author unknown)

If you trap the moment before its ripe
The tears of repentance you'll certainly wipe
But if once you let the ripe moment go
You can never wipe off the tears of woe.

William Blake (1757–1827)

But in history, as in travelling, men usually see
only what they already had in their own minds;
and few learn much from history, who do not bring
much with them to its study.

John Stuart Mill (1806–73)

I am quite my own master, agreeably lodged, perfectly easy in my circumstances. I am contented with my situation, and happy because I think myself so.

Alain Le Sage (1668–1747)

Dost thou love life, then do not squander time, for that is the stuff life is made of.

Benjamin Franklin (1706–90)

Trust no future howe'er pleasant!
Let the dead past bury its dead!
Act, act in the living present!
Heart within and God o'erhead!

Henry Wadsworth Longfellow (1807–82)

Tomorrow do thy worst,
  for I have lived today.

John Dryden (1631–1700)

Tomorrow cheats us all. Why dost thou stay,
And leave undone what should be done today?
Begin – the present minutes in thy power.

Thomas Hughes (1822–96)

Tomorrow to fresh woods and pastures new.

John Milton (1608–74)

Remembrance wakes with all her busy train,
Swells at my breast, and turns the past to pain.

Oliver Goldsmith (1728–74)

The Future, the Past, and the Here and Now ❀

Truth is brought to light by time.

Cornelius Tacitus (c.55–117)

Alas! Regardless of their doom,
The little victims play;
No sense have they of ills to come,
Nor care beyond today.

Thomas Gray (1716–71)

Well, Sir Anthony, since you desire it we will not anticipate the past; so mind, young people, our introspection will now be all to the future.

Richard Sheridan (1751–1816)

Learn, and think for yourself, is reasonable advice for the day; but let not the business of the day be so done as to prejudice the work of the morrow.

John Stuart Mill (1806–73)

The thing that hath been, it is that which shall be; and that which is done, is that which shall be done; and there is no new thing under the sun.

The Bible, Ecclesiastes 1:9

For what are men who grasp at praise sublime,
But bubbles on the rapid stream of time,
That rise and fall, that swell and are no more,
Born and forgot, ten thousand in an hour.

Edward Young (1683–1765)

Let us not burden our remembrances with
A heaviness that's gone.

William Shakespeare (1564–1616)

Seek not to know what must not be reveal'd;
Joys only flow where Fate is most conceal'd;
Too busie Man wou'd find his Sorrows more;
If future Fortunes he shou'd know before;
For by that knowledge of his Destiny
He would not live at all, but always die.

John Dryden (1631–1790)

Gather ye rose-buds while ye may,
Old time is still a-flying;
And this same flower which smiles today,
Tomorrow will be dying.

Robert Herrick (1591–1674)

. . . for whatever we may think or affect to think of the present age, we cannot get out of it . . . and, to be either useful or at ease, we must even partake its character . . . And since every age contains in itself the germ of all future ages as surely as the acorn contains the future forest, a knowledge of our own age is the fountain of prophecy.

John Stuart Mill (1806–73)

Happy the man, and happy he alone
He who can call today his own:
He who, secure within, can say,
Tomorrow do thy worst, for I have lived
    today.
Be fair or foul or rain or shine
The joys I have possessed, in spite of
    fate, are mine.
Not Heaven itself upon the past has
    power,
But what has been, has been,
    and I have had my hour.

John Dryden (1631–1700)

The men of the past, are those who continue to insist upon our still adhering to the blind guide. The men of the present, are those who bid each man look about for himself, with or without the promise of spectacles to assist him.

John Stuart Mill (1806–73)

Every day is the best day in the year. No man has learned anything rightly until he knows that every day is Doomsday.

Ralph Waldo Emerson (1803–82)

Was, and is, and will be, are but 'is'.

Alfred, Lord Tennyson ((1809–92)

We are always looking into the future,
but we see only the past.

Anne-Sophie Swetchine (1782–1857)

We all complain of the shortness of time, and yet have much more than we know what to do with. Our lives are spent either in doing nothing at all, or in doing nothing to the purpose, or in doing nothing that we ought to do; we are always complaining our days are few, and acting as though there would be no end of them.

Lucius Seneca (c. 4BC–AD65)

Employ thy time well if thou meanest to gain leisure, and, since you are not sure of a minute, throw away not an hour.

Benjamin Franklin (1706–90)

They usually resolve that the new light which has broken in upon them shall be the sole light; and they wilfully and passionately blew out the ancient lamp, which, though it did not show them what they now see, served very well to enlighten the objects in its immediate neighbourhood.

John Stuart Mill (1806–73)

That which hath been is now: and that
which is to be hath already been.

The Bible

Time is but a stream I go a-fishing in. I drink at it;
but while I drink I see the sandy bottom, and
detect how shallow it is. Its thin current slides
away, but eternity remains. I would drink deeper,
fish in the sky, whose bottom is pebbly with stars.

Henry David Thoreau (1817–62)

Time is a continual over-dropping of moments, which fall down one upon the other and evaporate.

Jean Paul (1763–1825)

The present time, youngest-born of eternity, child and heir of all the past times with their good and evil, and parent of all the future, is ever a new era to the thinking man.

Thomas Carlyle (1795–1881)

It is with history as it is with nature, as it is with everything profound, past, present, or future: the deeper we earnestly search into them, the more difficult are the problems that arise. He who does not fear them but boldly confronts them, will, with every step or advance, feel himself both more at his ease and more highly educated.

Johann Wolfgang von Goethe (1749–1832)

The future comes on slowly, the present flies like an arrow, the past stands still for ever.

Johann Schiller (1759–1805)

The present is the only reality and
the only certainty.

Arthur Schopenhauer (1788–1860)

O my People! This life of the present is
nothing but (temporary) convenience: it is
the Hereafter that is the Home that will last.'

The Qu'ran 40:39

In rivers, the water that you touch is the last of what has passed and the first of that which comes; so with time present.

Leonardo da Vinci (1452–1519)

O that I were where I would be!
Then should I be where I am not;
But where I am, there I must be,
And where I would be I can not.

Author Unknown

Be not the slave of our own past – plunge into the sublime seas, dive deep, and swim far, so you shall come back with self-respect, with new power, with an advanced experience, that shall explain and overlook the old.

Ralph Waldo Emerson (1803–82)

To find fault with our ancestors for not having annual parliaments, universal suffrage, and vote by ballot, would be like quarrelling with the Greeks and Romans for not using steam navigation . . . which would be, in short, simply finding fault with the third century before Christ for not being the eighteenth century after.

John Stuart Mill (1806–73)

'Verily, the knowledge of the Hour is with Allah (alone). It is He Who sends down rain, and He Who knows that is in the wombs. Nor does anyone know what it is that he will earn on the morrow; nor does anyone know in what land he is to die. Verily, with Allah is full knowledge and He is acquainted with (all things).

The Qu'ran 31:34

Take therefore no thought for the morrow: for the morrow shall take thought for the things of itself. Sufficient unto the day is the evil thereof.

The Bible, Jesus, Matthew 6:34

Mankind are then divided, into those who are still what they were, and those who have changed: into the men of the present age, and the men of the past. To the former, the spirit of the age is a subject of exultation; to the latter, of terror; to both, of eager and anxious interest.

John Stuart Mill (1806–73)

He answered and said unto them, When it is evening, ye say, It will be fair weather: for the sky is red. And in the morning, It will be foul weather to day, for the sky is red and lowring. O ye hypocrites, ye can discern the face of the sky, but can ye not discern the signs of the times?

The Bible, Jesus, Matthew 16:2–3

Lives of great men all remind us,
We can make our lives sublime;
And departing leave behind us
Footprints on the sands of time.

Henry Wadsworth Longfellow (1807–82)

Men must pursue things which are just in present, and leave the future to the Divine Providence.

Francis Bacon (1561–1626)

'Yes!' I answered you last night;
'No!' this morning, sir, I say:
Colours seen by candlelight
Will not look the same by day.

Elizabeth Barret Browning (1809–61)

A man should never be ashamed to own he
has been in the wrong, which is but saying,
in other words, that he is wiser today than
he was yesterday.

Jonathan Swift (1667–1745)

A great many things have been pronounced untrue and absurd, and even impossible, by the highest authorities in the age in which they lived, which have afterwards, within a very short period, been found to be both possible and true.

Catharine Crowe (c.1800–76)

Wait, thou child of hope, for time shall teach thee all things.

Martin Tupper (1810–89)

Time is at once the most valuable and the most perishable of all our possessions.

John Randolph (1773–1883)

Slow me down, Lord! Ease the pounding of my heart by the quieting of my mind. Steady my hurried pace with a vision of the eternal reach of time. Give me, amidst the confusion of my day, the calmness of the everlasting hills. Break the tension of my nerves and muscles with the soothing music of singing streams that live in my memory.

Author unknown

My name is Might-have-been:
I am also called No-more, Too-late, Farewell.

Dante Rossetti (1828–82)

In Relation to Others

Why, look you, how you storm!
I would be friends with you, and have your love.

William Shakespeare (1564–1616)

I was angry with my friend;
I told my wrath, my wrath did end.
I was angry with my foe:
I told it not, my wrath did grow

William Blake (1757–1827)

Always be ready to speak your mind,
    and a base man will avoid you.

William Blake (1757–1827)

His account of his other brother, a confectioner's household with two wives, was very curious. He and they, with his wife and sister-in-law, all live together, and one of the brother's wives has six children – three sleep with their own mother and three with their other mother – and all is quite harmonious.

Lucie Duff Gordon (1821–69)

Never can true reconcilement grow,
Where wounds of deadly hate have pierced
    so deep.

John Milton (1608–74)

It is easier to forgive an Enemy than to forgive a
    Friend:
The man who permits you to injure him, deserves
    your vengeance:

William Blake (1757–1827)

Two stars keep not their motion in one sphere.

William Shakespeare (1564–1616)

And why beholdest thou the mote that is in thy brother's eye, when thou thyself beholdest not the beam that is in thine own eye? Thou hypocrite; cast out first the beam out of thine own eye, and then shalt thou see clearly to pull out the mote that is in thy brother's eye.

The Bible, Jesus, Luke 6:21

I have tried to make friends by corporeal gifts
    but have only
Made enemies: I never made friends but by
    spiritual gifts;

William Blake (1757–1827)

Suppose I have committed a crime; forgive it. For, by Allah, how sweet is the beloved when he pardoneth!

The Thousand and One Nights

In early times, the great majority of the male sex were slaves, as well as the whole of the female. And many ages elapsed, some of them ages of high cultivation, before any thinker was bold enough to question the rightfulness, and the absolute social necessity, either of the one slavery or of the other.

John Stuart Mill (1806–73)

My mother bore me in the southern wild,
And I am black, but O! My soul is white;
White as an angel is the English child:
But I am black as if bereav'd of light.

William Blake (1757–1827)

Pardon thy brother when he mingles his right
    aiming with error;
And shrink from rebuking him if he swerve or
    decline;
Keep faith with him even though he fail in what
    thou and he have stipulated
And know that if thou seek a perfect man thou
    desirest beyond bounds

The Assemblies of Al–Hariri

Trust not a person in whose heart thou has made
    anger to dwell, nor think his anger hath ceased.
Verily, the vipers, which are smooth to the touch,
    and shew graceful motions, hide mortal poison.

The Thousand and One Nights

People are not aware how entirely, in former ages,
the law of superior strength was the rule of life;
how publicly and openly it was avowed . . . History
gives a cruel experience of human nature, in
showing how exactly the regard due to the life,
possessions, and entire earthly happiness of any
class of persons was measured by what they had
the power of enforcing . . .

John Stuart Mill (1806–73)

Forgiveness to the injured does belong.

John Dryden (1631–1700)

Blest be that spot, where cheerful guests retire
To pause from toil, and trim their evening fire;
Blest that abode, where want and pain repair,
And every stranger finds a ready chair;
Blest be those feasts with simple plenty crown'd,
Where all the ruddy family around
Laugh at the jests or pranks that never fail;
Or sigh with pity at some mournful tale;
Or press the bashful stranger to his food,
And learn the luxury of doing good.

Oliver Goldsmith (1728–74)

Forgive us our trespasses, as we forgive them that trespass against us.

The Bible, Jesus, The Lords Prayer

Be to her virtues very kind;
Be to her faults a little blind.

Matthew Prior (1664–1721)

Whate'er the passion, knowledge, fame, or pelf,
Not one will change his neighbour with himself.

Alexander Pope (1688–1744)

I think I could turn and live with animals, they
    are so placid and self-contain'd,
I stand and look at them long and long.
They do not sweat and whine about their
    condition.
They do not lie awake in the dark and weep for
    their sins,
They do not make me sick discussing their
    duty to God,
Not one is dissatisfied, not one is demented
    with the mania of owning things,
Not one kneels to another, nor to his kind that
    lived thousands of years ago,
Not one is respectable or unhappy over the
    whole earth.

Walt Whitman (1819–92)

It is by discussion also, that true opinions are discovered and diffused . . . All the inconsistencies of an opinion itself, with obvious facts, or even with other prejudices, discussion evolves and makes manifest . . .

John Stuart Mill (1806–73)

Backbite not, lest thou be backbitten; for probably, of him who saith a thing, the like will be said; And abstain from shameful words; utter them not when thou speakest seriously or when thou jestest.

The Thousand and One Nights

I'll not listen to reason . . . Reason always means
what someone else has got to say.

Elizabeth Gaskell (1810–65)

What law have I broken? Is it wrong for me to love
my own? Is it wicked for me because my skin is
red? Because I am Sioux; because I was born where
my fathers lived; because I would die for my people
and my country?

Tatanka Iyotake (c.1831–90)

But was there ever any domination which did not appear natural to those who possessed it?

John Stuart Mill (1806–73)

There is nothing in the whole world so painful as feeling that one is not liked. It always seems to me that people who hate me must be suffering from strange form of lunacy.

Sei Shonagon (c.966–1013)

People wish their enemies dead – but I do not: I say give them the gout, give them the stone!

Lady Mary Wortley Montague (1689–1726)

If something pleasant happens to you, don't forget to tell it to your friends, to make them feel bad.

Comte de Montrond (1768–1843)

Punishment is not for revenge, but to lessen crime and reform the criminal.

Elizabeth Fry (1780–1845)

We do not correct the man we hang;
we correct others by him.

Michel de Montaigne (1533–92)

When the people do not fear death, to what purpose is death still used (as a punishment) to overawe them? And should the people be kept in continual fear of death . . . ?

Lao Tsze (c.604–531 BC)

But indeed if any show patience and forgive, that would truly be an exercise of courageous will and resolution in the conduct of affairs.

The Qu'ran 43:43

Standing, as I do, in view of God and eternity, I realise that patriotism is not enough. I must have no hatred or bitterness towards anyone.

Edith Cavell (1865–1915)

Lord, make me an instrument of your peace
Where there is hatred let me sow love.

Prayer of St Francis (1181–1226)

I, young in life, by seeming cruel fate
Was snatch'd from Afric's fancied happy seat;
What pains excruciating must molest,
What sorrows labour in my parent's breast?
Steeled was that soul, and by no misery moved
That from a father seized his babe beloved:
Such, such my case, and can I then but pray
Others may never feel tyrannic sway?

Phillis Wheatley (*c.*1753–1784)

How say that by law we may torture and chase
A woman whose crime is the hue of her face?

Frances Ellen Watkins Harper (1825–1911)

Here is found liberty in the full sense of the word, liberty for the stranger within her gates, irrespective of race or creed, liberty and justice for all.

Susie King Taylor (1848–1912)

We are members of one great body. Nature planted in us a mutual love, and fitted us for a social life. We must consider that we were born for the good of the whole.

Lucius Seneca (c.4BC–AD65)

Moreover, not only towards the Jews, but towards all oriental peoples with whom we English come in contact, a spirit of arrogance and contemptuous dictatorialness is observable which has become a national disgrace to us.

George Eliot (1819–90)

All colours will agree in the dark.

Francis Bacon (1561–1626)

Digressions in a book are like foreign troops in a state, which argue the nation to want a heart and hands of its own; and often either subdue the natives, or drive them into the most unfruitful corners.

Jonathan Swift (1667–1745)

Each heart is a world. You find all within yourself that you find without. The world that surrounds you is the magic glass of the world within you.

Johann Lavater (1741–1801)

Mrs Williams was a kind-hearted good woman, and she treated all her slaves well. She had only one daughter, Miss Betsey, for whom I was purchased, and who was about my own age . . . This was the happiest period of my life; for I was too young to understand rightly my condition as a slave, and too thoughtless and full of spirits to look forward to the days of toil and sorrow.

Mary Prince (*c.*1788–1833)

Eyes speak all languages; wait for no letter of introduction; they ask no leave of age or rank; they respect neither poverty nor riches, neither learning, nor power, nor virtue, nor sex, but intrude and come again, and go through and through you in a moment of time.

Ralph Waldo Emerson (1803–82)

Four hostile newspapers are more to be feared than a thousand bayonets.

Napoleon Bonaparte (1769–1821)

Friendship is two souls in one body.

Author Unknown

Friendship is the shadow of the evening, which strengthens with the setting of the sun.

Jean de La Fontaine (1621–95)

No wise man can have a contempt for the prejudices of others; and he should even stand in a certain awe of his own, as if they were aged parents and monitors. They may in the end prove wiser than he.

William Hazlitt (1778–1830)

If we could read the secret history of our enemies, we should find in each man's life sorrow and suffering enough to disarm all hostility.

Henry Wadsworth Longfellow (1807–82)

Each man sees over his own experience a certain stain of error, whilst that of other men looks fair and ideal.

Ralph Waldo Emerson (1803–82)

We do not judge men by what they are in themselves, but by what they are relatively to us.

Anne-Sophie Swetchine (1782–1857)

Friendship is to be purchased only by friendship. A man may have authority over others; but he can never have their heart but by giving his own.

Bishop Thomas Wilson (1663–1755)

If one be himself devoid of uprightness, the upright will become crafty, the good will become depraved. Verily, mankind have been under delusion for many a day.

Therefore the sage is himself strictly correct, but does not cut and carve other people. He is chaste, but does not chasten others. He is straight, but does not straighten others. He is enlightened, but does not dazzle others.

Lao Tsze (c.604–531BC)

As a beauty I am not a star,
There are others more handsome by far.
But my face, I don't mind it,
For I keep behind it;
It's the people in front get the jar.

Thomas Woodrow Wilson (1856–1924)

But if the enemy incline towards peace,
do thou (also) incline towards peace . . .

The Qu'ran 8:61

. . . but whosoever shall smite thee on they right cheek, turn to him the other also.

And if any man will sue thee at the law, and take away thy coat, let have thy cloak also.

And whosoever shall compel thee to go a mile, go with him twain.

Give to him that asketh thee, and from him that would borrow thee turn not thou away.

The Bible, Jesus, Matthew 5:39–43

. . . nor defame nor be sarcastic to each other, nor call each other by (offensive) nicknames: ill-seeming is a name connoting wickedness (to be used of one) after he has believed: and those who do not desist are (indeed) doing wrong.

The Qu'ran 49:11

He that hath a satirical vein, as he maketh others afraid of his wit, so he had need be afraid of others memory.

Francis Bacon (1561–1626)

When the world has many prohibitory enactments, the people become more and more poor. When the people have many warlike weapons, the government gets into trouble.

Lao Tsze (c.604–531BC)

As long as war is regarded as wicked, it will always have its fascination. When it is looked upon as vulgar, it will cease to be popular.

Oscar Wilde (1854–1900)

Blessed are the peacemakers, for they shall be called the children of God.

The Bible, Jesus, Matthew 5:9

And since quietness is also lowliness, therefore a great kingdom by lowliness towards a small kingdom, may take that small kingdom. And a small kingdom, by lowlinesss toward a great kingdom, may take that great kingdom.

Lao Tsze (*c.*604–531BC)

The time will come when man
Will be as free and equal as the waves,
That seem to jostle, but that never jar.

Alfred Austin (1835–1913)

When a (courteous) greeting is offered you,
meet it with a greeting still more courteous,
or (at least) of equal courtesy.

The Qu'ran 4:86

It is not the life that passeth through the
mind, but the lie that sinketh in, and settleth
in it, that doth the hurt.

Francis Bacon (1561–1626)

All punishment is mischief. All punishment in itself is evil. Upon the principle of utility, if it ought at all to be admitted, it ought only to be admitted in as far as it promises to exclude some greater evil.

Jeremy Bentham (1748–1832)

Force is not a remedy.

John Bright (1811–89)

Of all the weak things in the world, nothing exceeds water: and yet of those who attack hard and strong things, I know not what is superior to it. Don't make light of this. The fact that the weak can conquer the strong, and the tender the hard, is known to all the world, yet none can carry it out in practice.

Lao Tsze (c.604–531BC)

Think when you are enraged with anyone, what would probably become your sentiments should he die during the dispute.

William Shenstone (1714–63)

No man can justly censure or condemn another, because indeed no man truly knows another.

Sir Thomas Browne (1605–1682)

What right have we to believe Nature under any obligation to do her work by means of complete minds only? She may find an incomplete mind a more suitable instrument for a particular purpose. It is the work that is done, and the quality in the worker by which it was done, that is alone of moment; and it may be of no great matter from a cosmical standpoint, if in other qualities of character he was singularly defective – if indeed he were hypocrite, adulterer, eccentric, or lunatic.

Henry Maudsley (1835–1918)

The sanest and best of us are of one clay with
lunatics and prison inmates, and death finally runs
the robustest of us down.

William James (1842–1910)

If things are ever to move upward, some one must
be ready to take the first step, and assume the risk
of it. No one who is not willing to try charity, to try
non-resistance . . . can tell whether these methods
will or will not succeed. When they do succeed,
they are far more powerfully successful than force
or worldly prudence.

William James (1842–1910)

Pray you use your freedom,
And, so far as you please, allow me mine
To hear you only; not to be compelled
To take your moral potions.

Philip Massenger (1583–1640)

. . . I say to you, love your enemies, bless
them that curse you, do good to them that
hate you, and pray for them which
despitefully use you, and persecute you:

The Bible, Jesus, Matthew 5:44

I have learned to see in all men, even in those most criminal, even in those from whom I have most suffered, undeveloped brothers to whom I owed assistance, love and forgiveness.

Author unknown

In nature there are neither rewards nor punishments – there are consequences.

Robert Ingersoll (1833–99)

About six or seven o'clock I walk out into a common that lies hard by the house, where a great many young wenches keep sheep and cows and sit in the shade singing ballads. I talk to them, and find they want nothing to make them the happiest people in the world, but the knowledge that they are so.

Dorothy Osborne (1627–95)

If a man should conquer in battle a thousand and a thousand more, and another man should conquer himself, his would be the greater victory, because the greatest of victories is the victory over oneself.

The Dhammapada

I wish that very one of us had come to such a state that even when we see the vilest of human beings we can see the God within, and instead of condemning, say, 'Rise, thou effulgent One, rise, thou who are always pure, rise thou birthless and deathless, rise almighty, and manifest your nature'.

Swami Vivekananda (1863–1902)

In Times of Trouble

I have a silent sorrow here;
A grief I'll ne'er impart;
It breathes no sigh, it sheds not tear,
But it consumes my heart.

Author unknown

Let the slave grinding at the mill run out into the
    field
Let him look up into the heavens and laugh in the
    bright air
Let the enchain'd soul shut up in darkness and in
    sighing
Whose face has never seen a smile in thirty weary
    years
Rise and look out his chains are loose his
    dungeon doors are open

William Blake (1757–1827)

Time consists of two days; this, bright; and that,
  gloomy;
And life, of two moieties; this safe; and that fearful.
Say to him who hath taunted us on account of
  misfortunes,
Doth fortune oppose any but the eminent?
Dost thou not observe that corpses float upon the
  sea,
While the precious pearls remain in its furthest
  depths?
When the hands of time play with us, misfortune is
  imparted to us by its protracted kiss.

The Thousand and One Nights

To change one's life: start immediately – do
it flamboyantly. No exceptions (no excuses).

William James (1842–1910)

When Fortune means to men most good,
She looks upon them with a threat'ning eye.

William Shakespeare (1564–1616)

I slept and dreamed that life was Beauty
I woke and found that life was Duty.
Was thy dream then a shadowy lie?
Toil on, poor heart, unceasingly;
And thou shalt find thy dream to be
A truth and noonday light to thee.

Ellen Sturgis Hooper (1816–41)

Go confidently in the direction of your dreams!
Live the life you've imagined. As you simplify your
life, the laws of the universe will be simpler;
solitude will not be solitude, poverty will not be
poverty, nor weakness weakness.

Henry David Thoreau (1817–62)

There is no duty we so much underrate as
the duty of being happy.

Robert Louis Stevenson (1850–94)

Be mild when thou art troubled by rage, and be
patient when calamity befalleth thee;
For the nights are pregnant with events, and give
birth to every kind of wonder.

The Thousand and One Nights

Where an equal poise of hope and fear
Does arbitrate the event, my nature is
That I incline to hope, rather than fear.

John Milton (1608–71)

Consider the doings of thy Lord, how happiness
cometh unto thee, with speedy relief;
And despair not when thou sufferest affliction; for
how many wondrous mercies attend affliction!

The Thousand and One Nights

'Tis time enough to bear a misfortune when
it comes, without anticipating it.

Lucius Seneca (c. 4BC–AD65)

In blackness, there is some virtue, if you observe
its beauty well, they eyes do not regard the white or
red. Were it not for the black of the mole on a fair
cheek, how would lovers feel the value of its
brilliancy? Were not musk black, it would not be
precious. Were it not for the black of night, the
dawn would not rise. Were it not for the black of
the eye, where would be its beauty? And thus it is,
the black ambergris has the purest fragrance.

Antar: A Bedouin Romance

In life's rough tide I sunk not down,
But swam till Fortune threw a rope,
Buoyant on bladders filled with hope.

Matthew Green (1696–1737)

The wretch condemn'd with life to part,
Still, still on hope relies,
And every pang that rends the heart
Bids expectation rise.
Hope, like the glimmering taper's light,
Adorns and cheers the way;
And still, as darker grows the night,
Emits a brighter ray.

Oliver Goldsmith (1728–74)

I can't sing. As a singist I am not a success. I am saddest when I sing. So are those who hear me. They are sadder even than I am.

Charles Farrer Browne (1836–68)

Where griping grefes the hart would wounde,
And dolefulle dumps the mynd oppresse,
There musicke with her silver-sound
With spede is wont to send redress
Of troubled mynds, in every sore,
Swete musicke hath a salve in store,

Richard Edwards (c.1523–1566)

Jog on, jog on, the foot path way,
And merrily hent the stile-a:
A merry heart goes all the day,
Your sad tires in a mile-a.

William Shakespeare (1564–1616)

How poor are they that have not patience!
What wound did ever heal but by degrees?

William Shakespeare (1564–1616)

Sublime virtue is profound, is immense, is
the reverse of everything else! It will bring
about a state of universal freedom.

Lao Tsze (*c.*604–531BC)

Not rural sights alone, but rural sounds
Exhilarate the spirit, and restore
The tone of languid nature.

William Cowper (1731–1800)

A sunbeam passes through
pollution unpolluted.

Eusebius (264–340)

Shadow owes its birth to light.

John Gay (1685–1732)

Blessed be he who first invented sleep; it covers a man all over like a cloak.

Miguel de Cervantes (1547–1616)

O Sleep, O gentle sleep!
Nature's soft nurse, how have I frighted thee,
That thou no more wilt weigh my eyelids down,
And steep my senses in forgetfulness?

William Shakespeare (1564–1616)

Tea! Thou soft, thou sober, sage, and venerable liquid . . . running, smile-smoothing, heart-opening, wink-tippling cordial, to whose glorious insipidity I owe the happiest moment of my life, let me fall prostrate.

Colley Cibber (1671–1757)

One pain is lessen'd by another's anguish;
One desperate grief cures with another's languish.

William Shakespeare (1564–1616)

Come unto me, all ye that labour and are heavy laden, and I will give you rest. Take my yoke upon you, and learn of me; for I am meek and lowly in heart and ye shall find rest unto your souls. For my yoke is easy, and my burden is light.

The Bible, Jesus, Matthew 11:28–30

To be, or not to be, that is the question;
Whether 'tis nobler in the mind, to suffer
The slings and arrows of outrageous fortune,
Or to take arms against a sea of troubles,
And, by opposing, end them?

William Shakespeare (1564–1616)

Care to our coffin adds a nail, no doubt;
And every grin so merry draws one out

John Wolcot (1738–1819)

O, what may man within him hide,
Though angel on the outward side.

William Shakespeare (1564–1616)

'Tis a truth well known to most
That whatsoever thing is lost;
We seek it, ere it come to light,
In every cranny but the right.

William Cowper (1731–1800)

Of what a strange nature is knowledge! It clings to the mind, when it has once seized on it, like a lichen on the rock.

Mary Shelley (1797–1851)

Almost spent, as I was, by fatigue, and the dreadful suspense I endured for several hours, this sudden certainty of life rushed like a flood of warm joy to my heart, and tears gushed from my eyes.

How mutable are our feelings, and how strange is that clinging love we have of life even in the excess of misery!

Mary Shelley (1797–1851)

Better by far that you should forget and smile
Than that you should remember and be sad.

Christina Rossetti (1830–94)

When Righteousness declines, O Bharata!
When Wickedness is strong, I rise, from age
to age, and take visible shape, and move a
man with men, Succouring the good,
thrusting the evil back, and setting virtue on
her seat again.

Bhagavad Gita, Book 4

Your own desires [for the narrow path that leads to God] are in the brightest light, and you regard them as house guests, but this wordly concern [about the people entrusted to you] lies in shadows and you look on it as an intruder. You don't allow yourself to see that they belong together, and this is why you so frequently experience depression in your spirit.

Hildegard of Bingen (1098–1179)

Employment is Nature's physician, and is essential to human happiness.

Claudius Galen (131–201)

Evil, what we call evil, must ever exist while man exists: evil, in the widest sense we can give it, is precisely the dark, disordered material out of which man's free will has to create an edifice of order and good.

Thomas Carlyle (1795–1881)

Dost thou not see that what thou lovest and what
    thou hatest are conjoined?
And that the delight of long life is disturbed by
    the mixture of grey hairs?
And that the thorns appear upon the branches
    together with the fruit that is gathered?
Who is he that hath never done evil? And who
    hath done good alone?
If thou tried the sons of this age, thou wouldst
    find that most of them had erred.

The Thousand and One Nights

The acknowledgement of our weakness is
the first step towards repairing our loss.

Thomas à Kempis (1380–1471)

The path of sorrow, and that path alone,
Leads to the land where sorrow is unknown.

William Cowper (1731–1800)

The Lord is my shepherd: I shall not want.
He maketh me to lie down in green pastures; he
   leadeth me beside the still waters.
He restoreth my soul: he leadeth me in the paths
   of righteousness for his name's sake.
Yea, though I walk through the valley of the
   shadow of death, I will fear no evil: for thou
   art with me; thy rod and thy staff they comfort
   me.

The Bible, Psalm 23

No order or profession of men is so sacred, no place so remote or solitary, but that temptations and troubles will find them out and intrude upon them.

Thomas à Kempis (1380–1471)

It is the height of folly to throw up attempting because you have failed. Failures are wonderful elements in developing the character.

Author Unknown

The difficult things in the world must all originate in what is easy: and the great things in the world must all originate in what is small. Therefore the sage never attempts what is great, and hence he is able to accomplish great things.

Lao Tsze (c.604–531BC)

The presence of the wretched is a burden to the happy: and alas! The happy still more so to the wretched.

Johann Wolfgang von Goethe (1749–1832)

People undertake things, and always fail when they are on the point of succeeding. If they were as careful of the end as they usually are of the beginning there would be no failures.

Lao Tsze (c.604–531BC)

Success is to be measured not so much by the position that one has reached in life as by the obstacles which he has overcome.

Booker T. Washington (1858–1915)

Come, blessed sleep, most full, most perfect, come:
Come, sleep, if so I may forget the whole;
Forget my body and forget my soul,
Forget how long life is and troublesome.

Christina Rossetti (1830–94)

I lay there . . . trying to go to sleep, but the harder I tried the wider awake I grew . . . My mind got a start by and by, and began to consider the beginning of every subject which has ever been thought of, but it never went further than the beginning: it was touch and go; it fled from topic to topic with a frantic speed. At the end of an hour my head was in a perfect whirl, and I was dead tired, fagged out.

Mark Twain (1835–1910)

Much of what we call evil is due entirely to the way men take the phenomenon. It can so often be converted into a bracing and tonic good by a simple change of the sufferer's inner attitude from one of fear to one of fight . . . Since you make them evil or good by your own thoughts about them, it is the ruling of your thoughts which proves to be your principal concern.

William James (1842–1910)

I live in a constant endeavour to fence against the evils of life by mirth, being firmly persuaded that every time a man smiles – but so much more so when he laughs – it adds something to this Fragment of Life.

Laurence Sterne (1713–68)

Give me a man that is not dull,
When all the world with rifts is full;
But unamazed dares clearly sing,
Whenas the roof's a-tottering;
And, though it falls, continues still
Ticking the cittern with his quill.

Robert Herrick (1591–1674)

Damn braces! Bless relaxes!
I hate scarce smiles. I love laughing.

William Blake (1757–1827)

God is our refuge and strength, a very present help
in trouble.
Therefore will we not fear, though the earth be
removed, and though the mountains be carried
into the midst of the sea.

The Bible, Psalm 46

I waited patiently for the Lord; and he inclined
unto me, and heard my cry.
He brought me up also out of an horrible pit, out of
the miry clay, and set my feet upon a rock, and
established my goings.

The Bible, Psalm 40

Even if the doctor does not give you a year, even if he hesitates about a month, make one brave push and see what can be accomplished in a week.

Robert Louis Stevenson (1850–94)

There is no misery greater than discontent. There is no calamity more direful than the desire of possessing. Therefore the sufficiency of contentment is an everlasting sufficiency.

Lao Tsze (*c*.604–531BC)

To sit in the shade on a fine day and look upon verdure is the most perfect refreshment.

Jane Austen (1775–1817)

It is rarely seldom that I seek consolation
in the Flowin Bole.

Charles Farrer Browne (1836–68)

There is a state of mind, known to religious men, but to no others, in which the will to assert ourselves and hold our own has been displaced by a willingness to close our mouths and be as nothing in the floods and waterspouts of God. In this state of mind . . . the time for tension in our soul is over, and that of happy relaxation, of calm deep breathing, of an eternal present, with no discordant future to be anxious about, has arrived.

William James (1842–1910)

When all is done and said,
In the end you shall find,
He most of all doth bathe in bliss
That hath a quiet mind.

Thomas Vaux (1510–56)

Happiness! happiness! Religion is only one of the ways in which men gain that gift. Easily, permanently, and successfully, it often transforms the most intolerable misery into the profoundest and most enduring happiness.

William James (1842–1910)

I give a mind of perfect mood, whereby they draw
  to Me
And, all for love of them, within their darkened
  souls I dwell
And, with bright rays of wisdom's lamp, their
  ignorance dispel.

Bhagavad Gita, Book 10

If this room is full of darkness for thousands of
years, and you come in and begin to weep and
wail, 'Oh, the darkness', will the darkness vanish?
Bring the light in, strike a match, and light comes
in a moment. So what good will it do you to think
all your lives, 'Oh, I have done evil, I have made
many mistakes'? It requires no ghost to tell us that.

Swami Vivekananda (1863–1902)

How far that little candle throws its beams!
So shines a good deed in a naughty world.

William Shakespeare (1564–1616)

The Noble Truth of Suffering is this: Birth is
suffering; ageing is suffering; sickness is suffering;
death is suffering; sorrow and lamentation, pain,
grief and despair are suffering; association with
unpleasant is suffering; dissociation from pleasant
is suffering; not to get what one wants is suffering –
in brief, the five aggregates of attachment are
suffering.

Buddha (c.563–483BC)

No warmth, no cheerfulness, no healthful ease,
No comfortable feel in any member –
No shade, no shine, no butterflies, no bees
No fruits, no flowers, no leaves, no birds –
November!

Thomas Hood (1799–1845)

A sense of humour keen enough to show a man his own absurdities will keep him from the commission of all sins, nor nearly all, save those that are worth committing.

Samuel Butler (The Younger) (1835–1902)

Where is the laughter that shook the rafter?
Where is the rafter, by the way?

Thomas Aldrich (1836–1907)

If life were always merry
Our souls would seek relief
And rest from weary laughter
In the quiet arms of grief.

Henry van Dyke (1852–1933)

Deep the silence round us spreading
All through the night
Dark the path that we are treading
All through the night.
Still the coming day discerning,
By the hope within us burning,
To the dawn our footsteps turning,
All through the night.

Author Unknown

Of Men and Women

It is by no means established that the brain of a woman is smaller than that of a man. If it is inferred merely because a woman's bodily frame generally is of less dimensions than a man's, this criterion would lead to strange consequences. A tall and large-boned man must on this showing be wonderfully superior in intelligence to a small man, and an elephant or whale must prodigiously excel mankind.

John Stuart Mill (1806–73)

'Tis better to have loved and lost
Than never to have loved at all.

Alfred Lord Tennyson (1809–92)

He loves to sit and hear me sing,
Then, laughing, sports and plays with me;
Then stretches out my golden wing,
And mocks my loss of liberty.

William Blake (1757–1827)

Let the eagle change his plume,
The leaf its hue, the flower its bloom;
But ties around his heart were spun
That could not, would not, be undone.

Thomas Campbell (1777–1844)

Her skin is like silk, and her speech is soft,
  neither redundant nor deficient;
Her eyes, God said to them, Be – and they were,
  affecting men's hearts with the potency of
  wine.
May my love for her grow more warm each night,
  and cease not until the day of judgment!

The Thousand and One Nights

Verily I wonder – but how full is love of wonders;
accompanied by anxieties and ardour and passion!

The Thousand and One Nights

I have lost my existence among mankind since your absence; for my heart loveth none but you.
Take my body, then, in mercy, to the place where you are laid; and there bury me by your side;
And if, at my grave, you utter my name, the moaning of my bones shall answer to your call.

The Thousand and One Nights

The world has never yet seen a truly great and virtuous nation, because in the degradation of woman the very fountains of life are poisoned at their source.

Lucretia Mott (1793–1880)

We hold these truths to be self-evident: that all men and women are created equal . . .

Elizabeth Stanton (1815–1902)

Women are supposed to be very calm generally. But women feel just as men feel; they need exercise for their faculties, and a field for their efforts, as much as they brothers do; they suffer from too rigid a restraint, too absolute a stagnation, precisely as men would suffer; and it is narrow-minded in their more privileged fellow-creatures to say that they ought to confine themselves to making puddings and knitting stockings, to playing on the piano and embroidering bags.

Charlotte Brontë (1816–55)

If civilisation is to advance at all in the future, it must be through the help of women, women freed of their political shackles, women with full power to work their will in society.

Emmeline Pankhurst (1857–1928)

I would earnestly ask my sisters to keep clear of both the jargons now current everywhere . . . of the jargon, namely about the 'rights' of women, which urges women to do all that men do . . . merely because men do it, and without regard to whether this is the best that women can do; and of the jargon which urges women to do nothing that men do, merely because they are women . . . Woman should bring the best she has, whatever that is . . . without attending to either of these cries.

Florence Nightingale (1820–1910)

The independence of women seemed rather less unnatural to the Greeks than to other ancients, on account of the fabulous Amazons (whom they believed to be historical) and the partial example afforded by the Spartan women; who, though no less subordinate by law than in other Greek states, were more free in fact, and being trained to bodily exercises in the same manner with men, gave ample proof that they were not naturally disqualified for them.

John Stuart Mill (1806–73)

She is the sun; her place is in heaven; comfort then the heart with a becoming patience
For thou art not able to ascend unto her; nor is she able to descend unto thee.

The Thousand and One Nights

Love keeps the cold out better than a cloak. It serves for food and raiment.

Henry Wadsworth Longfellow (1807–82)

Many a man thinks he understands women, because he has had amatory relations with several, perhaps with many of them. If he is a good observer, and his experience extends to quality as well as quantity, he may have learnt something of one narrow department of their nature – an important department, no doubt. But of all the rest of it, few persons are generally more ignorant, because there are few from whom it is so carefully hidden.

John Stuart Mill (1806–73)

Many waters cannot quench love, neither
can the floods drown it.

The Bible, Solomon's Song

Love, free as air, at sight of human ties,
Spreads his light wings, and in a moment flies.

Alexander Pope (1688–1744)

Love sought is good, but given
unsought is better.

William Shakespeare (1564–1616)

But love is blind, and lovers cannot see
The pretty follies that themselves commit

William Shakespeare (1564–1616)

Love, the sole disease thou canst not cure.

Alexander Pope (1688–1744)

What will not woman, gentle woman, dare,
When strong affection stirs her spirit up?

Robert Southey (1774–1843)

I should like to hear somebody openly enunciating the doctrine . . . 'It is necessary to society that women should marry and produce children. They will not do so unless they are compelled. Therefore it is necessary to compel them'. The merits of the case would then be clearly defined. It would be exactly that of the slaveholders of South Carolina and Louisiana.

John Stuart Mill (1806–73)

He is a fool, who thinks by force or skill
To turn the current of a woman's will.

Sir Samuel Tuke (c.1610–74)

The man who lays his hand upon a woman,
Save in the way of kindness, is a wretch
Whom 'twere gross flattery to name a coward.

John Tobin (1770–1804)

Men are men; the best sometimes forget.

William Shakespeare (1564–1616)

Sigh no more, ladies, sigh no more;
Men were deceivers ever;
One foot in sea, and one on shore,
To one thing constant never.

William Shakespeare (1564–1616)

Underneath this marble stone
Lie two beauties joined in one.
Two whose loves death could not sever;
For both lived, both died together.

Abraham Cowley (1618–67)

What a beard hast thou got! Thou has got more hair on thy chin than Dobbin my phill-horse has on its tail.

William Shakespeare (1564–1616)

Sir, you have the most insinuating manner, but indeed you should get rid of that odious beard – one might as well kiss a hedgehog.

Richard Sheridan (1751–1816)

What's female beauty but an air divine
Through which the mind's all gentle graces shine.

Edward Young (1683–1765)

'Tis not a lip, or eye, we beauty call,
But the joint force and full result of all.

Alexander Pope (1688–1744)

Where none admire, 'tis useless to excel;
Where none are beaux, 'tis vain to be a belle;
Beauty like wit, to judges should be shown;
Both most are valued where they best are known.

George Lyttelton (1709–73)

We never expected any love from one another, and
so we were never disappointed.

Richard Sheridan (1751–1816)

I do not wish them [woman] to have power over
men; but over themselves.

Mary Wollstonecraft (1759–97)

An English wife has no legal right even to her own clothes or ornaments; her husband may take them and sell them if he pleases, even though they be the gifts of relatives or friends, or bought before marriage.

Caroline Norton (1808–77)

. . . and ain't I a woman?
that little man in black there say
a woman can't have as much rights as a man
cause Christ wasn't a woman.
Where did your Christ come from?
From God and a woman!
Man had nothing to do with him!
If the first woman God ever made
was strong enough to turn the world
upside down, all alone,
together women ought to be able to turn it
rightside up again.

Sojourner Truth (c.1797–1883)

Now it is a curious consideration, that the only things which the existing law excludes women from doing, are the things which they have proved that they are able to do . . . Queen Elizabeth or Queen Victoria, had they not inherited the throne, could not have been entrusted with the smallest of the political duties . . .

John Stuart Mill (1806–73)

No golden weights can turn the scale
Of justice in His sight;
And what is wrong in woman's life
In man's cannot be right.

Frances Ellen Watkins Harper (1825–1911)

. . . that there is but one rule of right for the conduct of all rational beings; consequently that true virtue in one sex must be equally so in the other, whenever a proper opportunity calls for its exertion; and vice versa, what is vice in one sex, cannot have a different property when found in the other.

Catherine Macaulay (1731–91)

I always think that a man is one character to his wife, another to his family, another to her family, a fourth to a mistress . . . and so on, *ad infinitum*; but I think the wife, if they are happy and love each other, gets the pearl out of all the oyster shells.

Isabel Burton (1831–96)

'Tis a strange thing that women can't converse with a lawyer, a parson, nor a man midwife without putting them all to the same use, as if one could not sign a deed, say one's prayers, or take physic without doing you know what after it. This instinct is so odd, I am sometimes apt to think we were made to no other end. If that's true, lord ha' mercy upon me; to be sure, I shall broil in the next world for living in the neglect of a known duty in this.

Lady Mary Wortley Montagu (1689–1762)

Though we all day with care our work attend
Such is our fate, we know not when 'twill end
When evening's come, you homeward take your
    way;
We, 'till our work is done, are forced to stay.

Mary Collier (c.1690–1762)

I loathe myself today. I detest this woman who 'superintends' you and rushes about, slamming doors and slopping water – all untidy with her blouse out and her nails grimed. I am disgusted and repelled by the creature who shouts at you, 'You might at least empty the pail and wash out the tea leaves!'.

Katherine Mansfield (1888–1923)

As her husband, he may divorce her; as his wife the utmost 'divorce' she could obtain is permission to reside alone, married to his name. Marriage is a civil bond for him, an indissoluble sacrament for her.

Caroline Norton (1808–77)

O ye who believe! Let not some men among you laugh at others: it may be that the (latter) are better than the (former): nor let some women laugh at others: it may be that the (latter) are better than the (former);

The Qu'ran 49:11

You can conceive of nothing more interesting and curious than the conversation of a man learned and intelligent, and utterly ignorant of all our modern Western science.

Lucy Duff Gordon (1821–69)

I wish I were a man. If I were, I would be Richard Burton; but being only a woman, I would be Richard Burton's wife.

Isabel Burton (1831–96)

For lover's eyes more sharply sighted be
Than other men's, and in dear love's delight
See more than any other eyes can see.

Edmund Spenser (*c.*1552–99)

For it stirs the blood in an old man's heart,
And makes his pulses fly
To catch the thrill of a happy voice
And the light of a pleasant eye.

Nathaniel P. Willis (1806–67)

Fortune hath something of the nature of a woman, who, if she be too closely wooed, goes commonly the further off.

Charles V (1500–58)

The rhetoric of love is half-breath'd, interrupted words, languishing eyes, flattering speeches, broken sighs, pressing the hand, and falling tears: ah, how do they not persuade, how do they not charm and conquer.

Aphra Behn (1649–89)

It is only by mutual agreement and mutual yielding to one another that a happy marriage can be one.

Queen Victoria (1819–1901)

Women and men of retiring timidity are cowardly only in dangers which affect themselves, but the first to rescue when others are endangered.

Jean Paul (1763–1825)

Women know by nature how to disguise their emotions far better than the most consummate male courtiers can do.

William Thackeray (1811–63)

Marriage, by making us more contented,
causes us often to be less enterprising.

Christian Bovee (1820–1904)

To my very self I seemed imperious and
unreasonable; he smiled, betraying delight. Warm,
jealous and haughty, I knew not till now that my
nature had such a mood; he gathered me near his
heart. I was full of faults; he took them and me all
home. For the moment of utmost mutiny he
reserved the one deep spell of peace . . .

Charlotte Brontë (1816–55)

Jenny kiss'd me when we met;
Jumping from the chair she sat in;
Time, you thief! Who love to get
Sweets into your list, put that in.
Say I'm weary, say I'm sad;
Say that health and wealth have miss'd me;
Say I'm growing old, but add –
Jenny kiss'd me!

Leigh Hunt (1784–1859)

And among His Signs is this, that he created for you mates from among yourselves, that ye may dwell in tranquillity with them, and He has put love and mercy between your (hearts): verily, in that are Signs for those who reflect.

The Qu'ran 30:21

And the scribes and Pharisees brought unto him a woman taken in adultery; and when they had set her in the midst, they say unto him, Master, this woman was taken in adultery, in the very act. Now Moses in the law commanded us, that such should be stoned: but what sayest thou? . . . he . . . said unto them, He that is without sin among you, let him first cast a stone at her . . . When Jesus . . . saw none but the woman, he said unto her, Woman, where are those thine accusers? Hath no man condemned thee? She said, No man, Lord. And Jesus said unto her, Neither do I condemn thee; go, and sin no more.

The Bible, Jesus, John 8:3–11

There is a lady sweet and kind,
Was never face so pleased my mind:
I did but see her passing by,
And yet I love her till I die.

Author unknown

One should never trust a woman who tells
one her real age. A woman who would tell
one that, would tell one anything.

Oscar Wilde (1854–1900)

Saw a wedding in the church . . . and strange to see
what delight we married people have to see these
poor fools decoyed into our condition.

Samuel Pepys (1633–1703)

In marriage, a man becomes slack and selfish, and undergoes a fatty degeneration of his moral being.

Robert Louis Stevenson (1850–94)

Somewhere beneath the sun,
These quivering heart-strings prove it,
Somewhere there must be one
Made for this soul, to move it.

William Cory (1823–92)

If all men are born free, how is it that all women are born slaves?

Mary Astell (1688–1731)

That little man . . . he says women can't have as much rights as men, cause Christ wasn't a woman. Where did your Christ come from? From God and a woman. Man had nothing to do with him.

Sojourner Truth (c.1797–1883)

The female woman is one of the greatest institooshuns of which this land can boste.

Charles Farrer Browne (1836–68)

When a great kingdom takes a lowly position, it becomes the place of concourse for the world – it is the wife of the world. The wife by quietness invariably conquers the man.

Lao Tsze (c.604–531BC)

Why art thou silent and invisible
Father of Jealousy
Why dost thou hide thyself in clouds
From every searching Eye
Why darkness and obscurity
In all thy words and laws
That none dare eath the fruit but from
The wily serpents jaws
Or is it because Secresy
Gains females loud applause

William Blake (1757–1827)

Love ceases to be a pleasure when it
ceases to be a secret.

Aphra Behn (1640–89)

Alas, she married another. They frequently do. I
hope she is happy – because I am.

Charles Farrer Browne (1836–68)

There are wonders in true affection: it is a body of
enigmas, mysteries, and riddles; wherein two so
become one, as they both become two.

Sir Thomas Browne (1605–82)

What's the earth
With all its art, verse, music, worth –
Compared with love, found, gained, and kept?

Robert Browning (1812–89)

One should always be in love. That is the
reason one should never marry.

Oscar Wilde (1854–1900)

The fountains mingle with the river,
And the rivers with the ocean;
The winds of heaven mix for ever
With a sweet emotion;
Nothing in the world is single;
All things, by a law divine,
In one another's being mingle –
Why not I with thine?

Percy Bysshe Shelley (1792–1822)

To lovers I devise their imaginary world, with whatever they may need, as the stars of the sky, the red, red roses by the wall, the snow of the hawthorn, the sweet strains of music, or aught else they may desire to figure to each other the lastingness and beauty of their love.

The Hobos Will (written in 1898)

Men work and think, but women feel.

Christina Rossetti (1830–94)

Man has gone but little way; now he is waiting to see whether Woman can keep step with him; but instead of calling out, like a good brother, 'You can do it, if you only think so', or impersonally, 'any one can do what he tries to do', he often discourages with schoolboy brag: 'Girls can't do that; girls can't play ball.' But let anyone defy their taunts, break through and be brave and secure, they rend the air with shouts . . .

Margaret Fuller (1810–50)

An old man once courted me, hey dorum
darity
An old man once courted me, me being
young.
An old man once courted me,
Fain would he marry me –
'Ah maids, when you're young, never wed
an old man'

'For he's got no fal-lor-a-lum, fal-diddle
dor-a-lum
He's got no fal-lor-a-lum, fal-diddle all day,
He's got no fal-lor-a-lum, he's lost his ding-
dor-a-lum,
Ah maids, when you're young, never wed
an old man.'

Folk song (author unknown)

Says the mother to sweet sixteen, whom she would marry to a sixty-five-year-old money bag, 'Think what a thing it is to have a fine establishment; do be a reasonable being'.

Sarah Parton (1810–72)

For me, I neither know nor care
Whether a parson ought to wear
A black dress or a white dress;
I have a trouble of my own,
A wife who preaches in a gown
And lectures in a night dress.

Geoffrey Rose (1817–82)

If men are always more or less deceived on the subject of women, it is because they forget that they and women do not speak altogether the same language.

Henri Amiel (1828–81)

The vast mass of men have to depend on themselves alone; the vast mass of women hope or expect to get their life given to them.

William Bolitho (1890–1913)

Female and male God made the man.
His image is the whole, not half.

Coventry Patmore (1823–96)

Compassion and Caring

Though I speak with the tongues of men and of angels, and have not charity, I am become as sounding brass, or a tinkling cymbal. And though I have the gift of prophecy, and understand all mysteries, and all knowledge, and though I have all faith, so that I could remove mountains, and have not charity, I am nothing. And though I bestow all my goods to feed the poor, and though I give my body to be burned, and have not charity, it profiteth me nothing.

The Bible, St Paul, Corinthians 1:13

How sweet is the Shepherds sweet lot,
From the morn to the evening he strays:
He shall follow his sheep all the day
And his tongue shall be filled with praise.

For he hears the lamb's innocent call,
And he hears the ewe's tender reply,
He is watchful while they are in peace.
For they know their Shepherd is nigh.

William Blake (1757–1827)

Know ye not that the most precious of offerings is the relieving of sorrows, and the firmest cord of salvation is the importing to those who have need?

The Assemblies of Al-Hariri

Can I see another's woe
And not be in sorrow too.
Can I see another's grief,
And not seek for kind relief.

William Blake (1757–1827)

Blessed are they that mourn: for
they shall be comforted.

The Bible, Jesus, Matthew 5:4

An infant when it gazes on a light,
A child the moment when it drains the breast,
A devotee when soars the host in sight,
An Arab with a stranger for a guest,
A sailor when the prize has struck in fight,
A miser filling his most hoarded chest,
Feel rapture: but not such true joy are reaping,
As they who watch o'er what they love while
    sleeping.

Lord Byron (1788–1824)

When late I attempted your pity to move,
Why seem'd you so deaf to my prayer?
Perhaps it was right to dissemble your love,
But – why did you kick me down stairs?

Author unknown

That best portion of a good man's life,
His little nameless, unremembered acts of
   kindness and of love.

William Wordsworth (1770–1850)

The kiss of friendship, kind and calm,
May fall upon the brow like balm;
A deeper tenderness may speak
In precious pledges on the cheek;
Thrice dear may be, when young lips meet,
Love's dewy pressure, close and sweet;
But more than all the rest I prize
The faithful lips that kiss my eyes.

Elizabeth Chase Akers (1831–1911)

Who would not give a trifle to prevent
What he would give a thousand worlds to cure?

Edward Young (1683–1765)

To weep with them that weep doth ease some deal,
But sorrow flouted at is double death.

William Shakespeare (1564–1616)

Rejoice with them that do rejoice, and
weep with them that weep.

The Bible, Romans 12:15

Suppose a neighbour should desire
To light a candle at your fire,
Would it deprive your flame of light,
Because another profits by 't?

Robert Lloyd (1733–64)

For I am the only one of my friends
that I can rely upon.

Apollodorus (*second century*)

The man who melts with social sympathy,
though not allied,
Is of more worth than a thousand kinsmen

Euripides (*c.*484–406BC)

The lessons of prudence have charms
And slighted may lead to distress;
But the man whom benevolence warms
Is an angel who lives but to bless.

Robert Bloomfield (1766–1823)

In nature there's no blemish but the mind;
None can be called deformed but the unkind.

William Shakespeare (1564–1616)

On you be every bliss; and every day,
In home-felt joys delighted, roll away,
Yourselves, your wives, your long-descending race,
May every God enrich with every grace.

Alexander Pope (1688–1744)

My bounty is as boundless as the sea,
My love as deep, the more I give to thee
The more I have, for both are infinite.

William Shakespeare (1564–1616)

The kindest and the happiest pair
Will find occasion to forbear:
And something every day they live
To pity, and perhaps forgive.

William Cowper (1731–1800)

So many gods, so many creeds,
So many paths that wind and wind,
While just the art of being kind
Is all the sad world needs.

Ella Wheeler Wilcox (1855–1919)

I thought Love lived in the hot sunshine,
But O he lives in the moony light!
I thought to find Love in the heat of the day,
But sweet Love is the comforter of night.

Seek love in the pity of other's woe,
In the gentle relief of another's care,
In the darkness of night and the winter's snow,
In the naked and outcast, seek Love there.

William Blake (1757–1827)

For frequent tears have run the
colours from my life.

Elizabeth Barrett Browning (1806–61)

No people do so much harm as
those who go about doing good.

Mandell Creighton (1843–1901)

Altruism: the art of doing unselfish
things for selfish reasons.

Author unknown

Oh divine master,
Grant that I may not so much seek
To be consoled as to console
To be understood as to understand

Prayer of St Francis (1181–1226)

My heart throbbed with grief and terror so violently, that I pressed my hands quite tightly across my breast, but I could not keep it still, and it continued to leap as though it would burst out of my body. But who cared for that? Did one of the many bystanders . . . think of the pain that wrung the hearts of the negro woman and her young ones? No! No!

Mary Prince (c.1788–1834)

I had seen their tears and sighs, and I had heard their groans, and I would give every drop of blood in my veins to free them.

Harriet Tubman (c.1821–1913)

The sale began – young girls were there,
Defenceless in their wretchedness,
Whose stifled sobs of deep despair
Revealed their anguish and distress
And mothers stood with streaming eyes,
And saw their dearest children sold,
Unheeded rose their bitter cries,
While tyrants bartered them for gold.

Frances Ellen Watkins Harper (1825–1911)

Each good thought or action moves
The dark world nearer to the sun.

John Greenleaf Whittier (1807–92)

Generosity during life is a very different thing from generosity in the hour of death: one proceeds form genuine liberality and benevolence, the other from pride or fear.

Horace Mann (1756–1859)

Care is no cure, but rather a corrosive for things that are not to be remedied.

William Shakespeare (1564–1616)

Laugh, and the world laughs with you;
Weep, and you weep alone;
For the sad old earth must borrow its mirth
But has trouble enough of its own.

Ella Wheeler Wilcox (1855–1919)

Ingratitude and compassion never
cohabit the same breast.

Robert South (1634–1716)

It's the same the whole world over,
It's the poor wot gets the blame,
It's the rich wot gets the gravy.
Ain't it all a bleedin' shame?

Author unknown

Jesus said unto him, Thou shalt love the Lord thy
    God with all they heart, and with all thy soul,
    and with all thy mind.
This is the first and great commandment.
And the second is like unto it, Thou shalt love thy
    neighbour as thyself.

The Bible, Jesus, Matthew 22:37–39

If a madman were to come into this room with a stick in his hand, no doubt we should pity the state of his mind; but our primary consideration would be to take care of ourselves. We should knock him down first, and pity him afterwards.

Samuel Johnson (1709–84)

So give what is due to kindred, the needy, and the wayfarer. That is best for those who seek the Countenance of Allah, and it is they who will prosper.

The Qu'ran 30:38

Nobody can tell what I suffer! But it is always so. Those who do not complain are never pitied.

Jane Austen (1755–1817)

Momentarily considered, then, the saint may waste his tenderness and be the dupe and victim of his charitable fever, but the general function of his charity in social evolution is vital and essential. If things are ever to move upward, some one must be ready to take the first step, and assume the risk of it.

William James (1842–1910)

I expect to pass through this world but once;
any good thing therefore that I can do, or
any kindness that I can show to any fellow-
creature, let me do it now; let me not defer
or neglect it, for I shall not pass this way
again.

Attributed to Stephen Grellet (1773–1855)

If all the good people were clever,
And all clever people were good,
The world would be nicer than ever
We thought that it possibly could.
But somehow, 'tis seldom or never
The two hit it off as they should;
The good are so harsh to the clever,
The clever so rude to the good!

Elizabeth Wordsworth (1840–1932)

Those who spend their substance in the cause of Allah, and follow not up their gifts with reminders of their generosity or with injury – for them their reward is with their Lord: on them shall be no fear, nor shall they grieve.

The Qu'ran 2:262

Knowledge puffeth up, but charity edifieth.

The Bible, 1 Corinthians 8:1

The sage does not lay up treasures. The more he does for others, the more he has of his own. The more he gives to others, the more he is increased.

Lao Tsze (c.604–531BC)

Which now was of these three, thinkest thou, was neighbour unto him that fell among the thieves? And he said, He that shewed mercy on him. Then said Jesus unto him, Go, and do thou likewise.

The Bible, Jesus, Luke 10:36–37

. . . experience shows that there are times in every one's life when one can be bettter counseled by others than by one's self. Inability to decide is one of the commonest symptoms of ₁fatigued nerves; friends who see our troubles more broadly, often see them more wisely than we do; so it is frequently an act of excellent virtue to consult and obey a doctor, a partner, or a wife.

William James (1842–1910)

Withhold not good from them to whom it is due, when it is in the power of thine hand to do it. Say not unto they neighbour, Go, and come again, and tomorrow I will give; when thou has it by thee.

The Bible, Proverbs 3:27–28

Serve Allah, and join not any partners with Him; and do good – to parents, kinsfolk, orphans, those in need, neighbours who are near, neighbours who are strangers, the Companion by your side, the wayfarer (ye meet), and what your right hands possess: for Allah loveth not the arrogant, the vainglorious.

The Qu'ran 4:36

Pure and complete sorrow is as impossible as pure and complete joy.

Leo Tolstoy (1828–1910)

If I were a cassowary
On the plains of Timbuctoo,
I would eat a missionary,
Coat and bands and hymn-book too.

Attributed to Samuel Wilberforce (1805–1873)

By undivided attention to the passion-
nature, and increasing tenderness, it is
possible to be a little child.

Lao Tsze (c.604–531BC)

Compassion is that which is victorious in the attack and secure in the defence. When Heaven would save a man, it encircles him in compassion.

Lao Tsze (*c.*604–531BC)

I said, 'You must have been most miserable to be so cruel.'

Elizabeth Barrett Browning (1808–61)

He smarteth most who hards his smart,
And sues for no compassion.

Sir Walter Ralegh (*c.*1552–1618)

It is righteousness . . . to spend of your substance, out of love for Him, for your kin, for orphans, for the needy, for the wayfarer, for those who ask, and for the ransom of slaves; to be steadfast in prayer, and practise regular charity.

The Qu'ran 22:177

If you have any care for me, care for yourself.

Publius Ovid (43BC–AD17)

The gentle mind by gentle deeds is known.

Herbert Spencer (1820–1903)

Shall I seek for (my) Cherisher other than
Allah, when He is the Cherisher of all things
(that exist)? Every soul draws the meed of its
acts on none but itself: no bearer of burdens
can bear the burden of another.

The Qu'ran 6:164

For there is no friend like a sister
In calm or stormy weather;
To cheer one on the tedious way,
To fetch one if one goes astray,
To lift one if one totters down.
To strengthen whilst one stands.

Christina Rossetti (1830–94)

Plenty of people wish well to any good cause, but very few care to exert themselves to help it, and still fewer will risk anything in its support. 'Some one ought to do it, but why should I?' is the ever re-echoed phrase of weak-kneed amiability.

Annie Besant (1847–1933)

'Love your enemies!' Mark you, not simply those who happen not to be your friends, but your enemies, your positive and active enemies. Can there in general be a level of emotion so unifying, so obliterative of differences between man and man . . . they (the effects) might conceivably transform the world.

William James (1842–1910)

For hate is not conquered by hate: hate is conquered by love. This is a law eternal.

The Dhammapada

A certain man went down from Jerusalem to Jericho, and fell among thieves, which stripped him of his raiment, and wounded him, and departed, leaving him half dead . . .

But a certain Samaritan, as he journeyed, came where he was, and when he saw him, he had compassion on him. And went to him, and bound up his wounds, pouring in oil and wine, and set him on his own beast, and brought him to an inn, and took care of him . . .

The Bible, Jesus, Luke 10

All breathing, existing, living, sentient creatures should not be slain, nor treated with violence, nor abused, nor tormented, nor driven away. This is the pure, unchangeable, eternal law.

Jaina Sutra

Once it came into my heart, and whelmed me like
    a flood,
That these too are men and women, human flesh
    and blood;
Men with hearts and men with souls, though
    trodden down with mud.

Christina Rossetti (1830–94)

Whosoever on the night of the nativity of the young Lord Jesus, in the great snows, shall fare forth bearing . . . a wisp of hay for the shivering horse, a cloak of raiment for the stranded wayfarer . . . a garland of bright red berries for one who has worn chains, a dish of crumbs with a song of love for all huddled birds who thought that song was dead . . . to him shall be proffered and returned gifts of such an astonishment as will rival the hues of heaven, so that though he live to the great age when man goes stooping . . . yet shall he walk upright and remembering, as one whose heart shines like a great star in his breast.

Author unknown

Divinity and the Divine

There is surely a piece of Divinity in us, something that was before the elements, and owes no homage to the sun.

Sir Thomas Browne (1605–82)

If God did not exist, it would be necessary to invent him.

François Voltaire (1694–1778)

Let us weigh the gain and the loss in wagering that God is. Let us estimate the two chances. If you gain, you gain all; if you lose, you lose nothing. Wager then without hesitation that He is.

Blaise Pascal (1623–70)

One Force in every place, though manifold.
I am the Sacrifice. I am the Prayer.
I am the Funeral Cake set for the dead.
I am the healing herb. I am the ghee
The Mantra, and the flame, and that which burns.
I am, of all this boundless Universe,
The Father, Mother, Ancestor and Guard.

Bhagavad Gita, Book 9

And every Natural Effect has a Spiritual Cause,
    and Not
A Natural; for a Natural Cause only seems, it is a
    Delusion
Of Ulro: & a ratio of the perishing Vegetable
    Memory.

William Blake (1757–1827)

May the road rise to meet you
May the wind be always at your back
May the sun shine warm upon your face
The rain fall soft upon your field
And until we meet again
May God hold you in the hollow of his hand.

Irish Blessing

God be in my head, and in my understanding
God be in my eyes, and in my looking
God by in my mouth, and in my speaking
God be in my heart, and in my thinking
God be at my end, and at my departing.

Old Sarum Primer

The nature of infinity is this: That everything has
    its
Own Vortex; and when once a traveller thro
    Eternity.
Has passd that Vortex, he perceives it roll
    backward behind
His path, into a globe itself infolding; like a sun:
Or like a moon, or like a universe of starry
    majesty

William Blake (1757–1827)

Come to the edge, he said
They said: We are afraid.
Come to the edge, he said.
They came.
He pushed them . . . and they flew.

Guillaume Apollinaire (1880–1918)

I am the wind that breathes upon the sea
I am the wave on the ocean
I am the murmur of leaves rustling
I am the rays of the sun
I am the beam of the moon and stars
I am the power of trees growing
I am the bud breaking into blossom
I am the movement of the salmon swimming
I am the courage of the wild boar fighting
I am the speed of the stag running
I am the strength of the ox pulling the plough
I am the size of the mighty oak tree
And I am the thoughts of all people
Who praise my beauty and grace.

The Black Book of Carmarthen (*Twelfth Century*)

Before enlightenment – chop wood, carry water
After enlightenment – chop wood, carry water.

Zen Proverb

Three joints in the finger, but only one finger fair
Three leaves of the shamrock yet only one
    shamrock to wear
Frost, snowflakes and ice, yet all in water their
    origin share
Three Persons in God; to one God alone we make
    prayer.

Traditional Irish

The nature of the mind when understood
No human words can compass or disclose
Enlightenment is nought to be obtained
And he that finds it does not say he knows.

Edwin Arnold (1832–1904)

More things are wrought by prayer
Than this world dreams of.

Alfred, Lord Tennyson (1809–92)

God and Nature met in light.

Alfred, Lord Tennyson (1809–92)

A God alone can comprehend A God.

Author unknown

Filled was the air with a dreamy and magical
    light; and the landscape
Lay as if new created in all the freshness of
    childhood.
Peace seemed to lay upon earth, and the restless
    heart of the ocean
Was for a moment consoled. All sounds were in
    harmony blended.

Henry Wadsworth Longfellow (1807–82)

May the raindrops fall lightly on your brow
May the soft winds freshen your spirit
May the sunshine brighten your heart
May the burdens of the day rest lightly upon you
And may God enfold you in love.

Ancient Irish Prayer

This sacred shade and solitude, what is it?
Tis the felt presence of the Deity.
Few are the faults we flatter when alone:
By night an atheist half believes a God.

Edward Young (1683–1765)

Prayer moves the hand that moves the Universe.

Author Unknown

Lord of my heart

Give me vision to inspire me that, working or resting, I may always think of you.

Lord of my heart

Give me light to guide me that, at home or abroad, I may always walk in your way.

Lord of my heart

Give me wisdom to direct me that, thinking or acting, I may always discern right from wrong.

Heart of my own heart

Whatever befall me, rule over my thoughts and feelings, my words and actions.

Ancient Irish Prayer

I am positive I have a soul; nor can all the books with which materialists have pestered the world, ever convince me to the contrary.

Laurence Sterne (1713–68)

I am Alpha and Omega, the beginning and the end, the first and the last.

The Bible, Revelation 22:13

I speak of that learning which makes us acquainted with the boundless extent of nature, and the universe, and which even while we remain in this world, discovers to us both heaven, earth, and sea.

Marcus Tullius Cicero (106–43BC)

With devotion's visage,
And pious action, we do sugar o'er
The devil himself.

William Shakespeare (1564–1616)

Who can believe with common sense,
A bacon slice gives God offence;
Or, how a herring hath a charm
Almighty vengeance to disarm?
Wrapt in majesty divine,
Does he regard on what we dine?

Jonathan Swift (1667–1745)

Flower in the crannied wall,
I pluck you out of the crannies,
I hold you here, root and all, in my hand,
Little flower – but if I could understand
What you are, root and all, and all in all,
I should know what God and man is.

Alfred, Lord Tennyson (1809–92)

When there is no love, put love, and
there you will find love.

St John of the Cross (1542–91)

Make Thyself visible, Lord of all prayers. Show me
Thy very self, the Eternal God.

See ME! See what thou prayest!
Thou canst not! Nor with human eyes, Arjuna,
  ever mayest.
Therefore I give thee sense divine. Have other
  eyes, new light!
And look! This My glory, unveiled to mortal sight.

Bhagavad Gita, Book 11

I am a flame of fire, blazing with passionate love;
I am a spark of light, illuminating the deepest
    truth;
I am a rough ocean, heaving with righteous anger;
I am a calm lake, comforting the troubled breast;
I am a wild storm, raging at human sins;
I am a gentle breeze, blowing hope in the
    saddened heart;
I am dry dust, choking wordly ambition;
I am wet earth, bearing rich fruits of grace.

The Black Book of Carmarthen (*Twelfth Century*)

In the evening of life, we will be
judged on love alone.

St John of the Cross (1542–91)

Impenetrable,
Unentered, unassailed, unharmed, untouched,
Immortal, all-arriving, stable, sure,
Invisible, ineffable, by word
And thought unencompassed, ever all itself,
Thus is the Soul declared!

Bhagavad Gita, Book 2

End and Beginning are dreams!
Birthless and deathless and changeless remaineth
    the spirit for ever:
Death hath not touched it all, dead though the
    house of it seems!

Bhagavad Gita, Book 2

Nay, but as when one layeth his worn-out robes
   away,
And, taking new ones, sayeth, 'These will I wear
   to-day!'
So putteth by the spirit lightly its garb of flesh
And passeth to inherit a residence afresh.

Bhagavad Gita, Book 2

Of many thousand mortals, once, perchance,
Striveth for Truth; and of those few that strive –
Nay, and rise high – one only – here and there –
Knoweth Me as I am, the very Truth.

Bhagavad Gita, Book 7

The stars, the thoughts of
God in the Heavens.

Henry Wadsworth Longfellow (1807–82)

I am not known
To evil-doers, nor to foolish ones,
Nor to the base and churlish; nor to those
Whose mind is cheated by the show of things,
Nor those that take the way of beings of low
    nature.

Bhagavad Gita, Book 7

When the world has Tao, horses are used only for
    purposes of agriculture.
When the world has not Tao, war horses are bred
    on the waste common.

Lao Tsze (*c.*604–531 BC)

Four sorts of mortals know me; he who weeps,
Arjuna, and the man who yearns to know;
And he who toils to help; and he who sits
Certain of me, enlightened.

Bhagavad Gita, Book 7

Moreover, when a soul departeth, fixed
In Soothfastness, it goeth to the place,
Perfect and pure, of those that know all Truth.
If it departeth in set habitude
Of Impulse, it shall pass into the world
Of spirits tied to works; and if it dies
In hardened ignorance, that blinded soul
Is born anew in some unlighted womb

Bhagavad Gita, Book 14

Everywhere I am hindered of meeting God in my
brother, because he has shut his own temple
doors, and recites fables merely of his brother's or
his brother's brother's God.

Ralph Waldo Emerson (1803–82)

God's Spirit breathes and speaks: in wintertime, God takes care of the branch that is love. In summer, God causes that same branch to be green and to sprout with blossoms. God removes diseased outgrowths that could do harm to the branch.

Hildegard of Bingen (1098–1179)

Hard labor and unkindness was too much for me; in three months, my health and strength were gone. I often looked at my employers, and thought to myself, is this your religion? . . . They had family prayers, morning and evening. Oh! yes, they were sanctimonious!

Nancy Gardner Prince (*c.*1799–*unknown*)

Teach us dear Lord, to serve you as you
deserve to be served,
To give and not to count the cost
To fight and not to heed the wounds
To toil and not to ask for any reward
Save that of knowing that we do your will.

Prayer of St Ignatius of Loyola (1491–1556)

From within or behind, a light shines
through us upon things, and makes us aware
that we are nothing, but the light is all.

Ralph Waldo Emerson (1803–82)

And do, my dear, always remember to ask God for light and help – for with Him all things are possible – and it almost astonishes one sometimes to find how He sends down answers to one's prayers in new bright thoughts, or in even more bright and lovely peace.

Elizabeth Gaskell (1810–65)

Feeling is all: name is sound and smoke veiling heaven's splendour.

Johann Wolfgang von Goethe (1749–1832)

Thirty spokes unite in one nave, and by that part which is non-existent, it is useful for a carriage wheel. Earth is moulded into vessels, and by their hollowness they are useful as vessels. Doors and windows are cut out in order to make a house, and by its hollowness it is useful as a house.

So then existence may be said to correspond to gain, but non-existence to use.

Lao Tsze (c.604–531BC)

Thought disturbs the world, and thought
    of God
Unsettles most of all: for it is life,
And only life can comprehend its force,
Or guide it.

William Smith (1846–94)

Music is a kind of inarticulate unfathomable speech, which leads us to the edge of the infinite, and lets us for moments gaze into that.

Thomas Carlyle (1795–1881)

The problem of life is to make the ideal real, and convert the divine at the summit of the mountain into the human at its base.

Charles Parkhurst (1842–1933)

The present moment is a potent divinity.

Johann Wolfgang von Goethe
(1749–1832)

In the New Testament there is internal evidence that parts of it have proceeded from an extraordinary man; and that other parts are of the fabric of very inferior minds. It is as easy to separate those parts, as it is to pick out diamonds from dunghills.

Thomas Jefferson (1743–1826)

Truth has never been, can never be, contained in any one creed or system.

Mary Ward (1851–1920)

And our Lord opened my inner eye and showed my soul in the middle of my heart. The soul was as large as an infinite world and like a blessed kingdom.

Julian of Norwich (1313–*c.*1416)

Neither are the good good, nor the evil evil, nor is life life, nor death death . . . Thus one who hears the word 'God' does not perceive what is correct . . . So also with 'life' and 'light' and 'resurrection'.

Author unknown

All at once, without warning of any kind, I found myself wrapped in a flame-coloured cloud . . . Directly afterwards there came upon me a sense of exultation, of immense joyousness, accompanied or immediately followed by an intellectual illumination quite impossible to describe. Among other things, I did not merely come to believe, I saw that the universe is not composed of dead matter, but is, on the contrary, a living Presence; I became conscious in myself of eternal life. It was not a conviction that I would have eternal life, but a consciousness that I possessed eternal life then.

William James (1842–1910)

Allah is the Light of the heavens and the earth. The parable of His Light is as if there were a Niche and within it a Lamp: the Lamp enclosed in Glass; the glass as it were a brilliant star: lit from a blessed Tree, an Olive, neither of the East nor of the West, whose oil is well-nigh luminous, though fire scarce touched it: Light upon Light!

The Qu'ran 24:35

It is sown a natural body: it is raised a spiritual body. There is a natural body, and there is a spiritual body.

The Bible, 1 Corinthians 15:15

In Me are all existences contained;
Not I in them.

Bhagavad Gita, Book 9

The Truth comes from Allah alone;
so be not of those who doubt.

The Qu'ran 3:60

Be still, and know that I am God.

The Bible, Psalm 46

Ask, and it shall be given you; seek, and ye shall find; knock, and it shall be opened unto you:
For every one that asketh receiveth, and he that seeketh findeth; and to him that knocketh it shall be opened.

The Bible, Jesus, Matthew 7:7–8

Canst thou by searching find out God? canst thou find out the Almight unto perfection? It is as high as heaven; what canst thou do? deeper than hell, what canst thou do? The measure thereof is longer than the earth, and broader than the sea.

The Bible, Job 11:7–9

We have just enough religion to make us hate, but not enough to make us love one another.

Jonathan Swift (1667–1745)

Tao, in its passing out of the mouth, is weak and tasteless. If you look at it, there is nothing to fill the eye. If you listen to it, there is nothing to fill the ear. But if you use it, it is inexhaustible.

Lao Tsze (c.604–531BC)

We find great things are made of little things,
And little things go lessening, till at last
Comes God behind them.

Robert Browning (1812–89)

But God hath chosen the foolish things of the
   world to confound the wise; and God hath
   chosen the weak things of the world to
   confound the things which are mighty;
And base things of the world, and things which are
   despised, hath God chosen, yea, and things
   which are not, to bring to nought things that
   are.

The Bible, 1 Corinthians 1:26–29

The voice of the people has about it something of
the divine: for how otherwise can so many heads
agree together as one?

Francis Bacon (1561–1626)

Music . . . strikes in me a deep fit of devotion, and a profound contemplation of the First Composer. There is something in it of Divinity more than the ear discovers.

Sir Thomas Browne (1605–82)

And then, when the man neither careth for nor desireth anything but the eternal Good alone, and seeketh not himself nor his own things, but the honour of God only, he is made a partaker of all manner of joy, bliss, peace, rest, and consolation, and so the man is henceforth in the kingdom of heaven.

Theologica Germanica (Sixteenth century)

Geology, ethnology, what not? –
(Greek endings, each the little passing bell
that signifies some faith's about to die.)

Robert Browning (1812–89)

Lord, thou knowest what is best; let this or that be according as thou wilt. Give what thou wilt, so much as thou wilt, when thou wilt. Do with me as thou knowest best, and as shall be most to thine honour. Place me where thou wilt, and freely work thy will with me in all things.

Thomas à Kempis (1380–1471)

I believe a leaf of grass is no less than the journey
    work of the stars,
And the pismire is equally perfect, and a grain of
    sand, and the egg of a wren
And the tree toad is a chef d'oeuvre for the
    highest
And the running blackberry would adorn the
    parlours of heaven.

Walt Whitman (1819–92)

If there should rise
Suddenly within the skies
Sunburst of a thousand suns
Flooding earth with beams undeemed of,
Then might be that Holy One's Majesty and
    radiance dreamed of.

Bhagavad Gita, Book 11

In the beginning was the Word, and the Word was
with God, and the Word was God. The same
was in the beginning with God.
All things were made by him; and without him was
not anything made that was made.
In him was life; and the life was the light of men.
And the light shineth in darkness; and the
darkness comprehended it not.

The Bible, John 1:1–5

In mystical literature such self-contradictory
phrases as 'dazzling obscurity', 'whispering
silence', 'teeming desert', are continually met
with. They prove that not conceptual speech,
but music rather, is the element through
which we are best spoken to by mystical truth.

William James (1842–1910)

Every man whose heart is no longer shaken by any doubt, knows with certainty that there is no being save only One.

Muhammed Shabistari (*written* 1317)

This act is prayer, by which term I understand no vain exercise of words, no mere repetition of certain sacred formulae, but the very movement itself of the soul, putting itself in a personal relation of contact with the mysterious power of which it feels the presence – it may be even before it has a name by which to call it. Wherever this interior prayer is lacking, there is no religion . . .

William James (1842–1910)

He will forgive you your sins, and admit you to Gardens beneath which rivers flow, and to beautiful mansions in Gardens of Eternity: that is indeed the Supreme Achievement.

The Qu'ran 61:12

Moreover, something is or seems,
That touches me with mystic gleams,
Like glimpses of forgotten dreams –

Of something felt, like something here;
Of something done, I know not where;
Such as no language may declare.

Alfred, Lord Tennyson (1809–92)

Deep peace of the running wave to you
Deep peace of the silent stars
Deep peace of the flowing air to you
Deep peace of the quiet earth
May peace fill your soul
Let peace make you whole.

A Celtic Blessing

It is as if there were in the human consciousness a sense of reality, a feeling of objective presence, a perception of what we may call 'somewhere there', more deep and more general than of the special and particular 'senses' by which the current psychology supposes existent realities to be originally revealed.

William James (1842–1910)

Why does man go out to look for a God? . . . It is your own heart beating, and you did not know, you were mistaking it for something external.

Swami Vivekananda (1863–1902)

Passage through Life

My mother groan'd! My father wept.
Into the dangerous world I leapt:
Helpless, naked, piping loud;
Like a fiend hid in a cloud.

William Blake (1757–1827)

What you say of the pride of giving life to an immortal soul is very fine, dear, but I own I can not enter into that; I think much more of our being like a cow or a dog at such moments; when our poor nature becomes so very animal and unecstatic.

Queen Victoria (1819–1901)

Amongst the feathered race, whilst the hen keeps the young warm, her mate stays by to cheer her; but it is sufficient for man to condescend to get a child, in order claim it. – A man is a tyrant!

Mary Wollstonecraft (1759–97)

There is nothing better for a child
than its mother's milk.

The Thousand and One Nights

The child's murmuring is more and is less than words; there are no notes, and yet it is a song, there are no syllables, and yet it is language . . . This poor stammering is a compound of what the child said when it was an angel, and of what it will say when it becomes a man.

Victor Hugo (1802–85)

The tear down childhood's cheek that flows,
Is like the dewdrop on the rose;
When next the summer breeze comes by,
And waves the bush, the flower is dry.

Sir Walter Scott (1771–1832)

Know you what it is to be a child? It is to be something very different from the man of today. It is to have a spirit yet streaming from the waters of baptism; it is to believe in love, to believe in loveliness, to believe in belief; it is to turn pumpkins into coaches, and mice into horses, lowness into loftiness, and nothing into everything, for each child has its fairy godmother in its own soul; it is to live in a nutshell and to county yourself the king of infinite space;

It is to know not as yet that you are under sentence of life, nor petition that it be commuted into death.

Francis Thompson (1859–1907)

And first, I give to good fathers and mothers, but in trust for their children, nevertheless, all good little words of praise and all quaint pet names, and I charge said parents to use them justly, but generously, as the needs of their chidren shall require.

The Hobos Will (*written in* 1898)

The place is very well and quiet, and the children only scream in a low voice.

Lord Byron (1788–1824)

Childhood has no forebodings; but then it is soothed by no memories of outlived sorrow.

George Eliot (1819–80)

Children should have their times of being off duty, like soldiers.

John Ruskin (1819–1900)

The Imagination is not a State: it is the Human Existence itself.

William Blake (1757–1827)

The wisest doctor is gravelled by the inquisitiveness of a child.

Ralph Waldo Emerson (1803–82)

Let early education be a sort of amusement; you will then be better able to find out the natural bent.

Plato (427–347BC)

Confine not the education of your daughters to what is regarded as the ornamental parts of it, nor deny the graces to your sons.

Catherine Macaulay (1731–91)

'Do you know who made you?' 'Nobody, as I knows of,' said the child, with a short laugh. The idea appeared to amuse her considerably; for her eyes twinkled, and she added – 'I 'spect I growed. Don't think anybody ever made me.'

Harriet Beecher Stow (1812–96)

Children know
Instinctive taught, the friend and foe.

Sir Walter Scott (1771–1832)

Any system of religion that has any thing in it that shocks the mind of a child cannot be a true system.

Thomas Paine (1737–1809)

We cannot fashion our children after our fancy. We must have them and love them, as God has given them to us.

Johann Wolfgang von Goethe (1749–1832)

The Men! O what venerable and reverend creatures did the aged seem! Immortal Cherubims! And the young men glittering and sparkling Angels, and maids strange seraphic pieces of life and beauty! Boys and girls tumbling in the street, and playing, were moving jewels.

Thomas Traherne (1637–74)

Says the conservative father to his son, whom he would force into some profession or employment for which nature has utterly disqualified him, 'Are you wiser than your father? do be a reasonable being'.

Sarah Parton (1811–72)

Youth, enthusiasm, and tenderness are like the days of spring. Instead of complaining, O my heart, of their brief duration, try to enjoy them.

Friedrich Ruckert (1789–1866)

Youth will never live to age, without they keep themselves in breath with exercise, and in heart with joyfulness.

Sir Philip Sidney (1554–86)

Education does not mean teaching people to know what they do not know; it means teaching them to behave as they do not behave.

John Ruskin (1819–1900)

Education, however indispensable in a cultivated age, produces nothing on the side of genius. Where education ends, genius often begins.

Isaac Disraeli (1766–1848)

Education may work wonders as well in warping the genius of individuals as in seconding it.

Amos Bronson Alcott (1799–1888)

Nobody thinks it necessary to make a law that only a strong-armed man shall be a blacksmith. Freedom and competition suffice to make blacksmiths strong-armed men, because the weak-armed can earn more by engaging in occupations for which they are more fit.

John Stuart Mill (1806–73)

Do not follow where the path may lead.
Go, instead, where there is no path
And leave a trail.

Anonymous

Afoot and light-hearted I take to the open road
Healthy, free, the world before me,
The long brown path before me leading me
                              wherever I choose.

Walt Whitman (1819–92)

Life is like music; it must be composed by ear,
feeling and instinct, not by rule.

Samuel Butler (1835–1902)

The fates lead him who will – him
who won't they drag.

Lucius Seneca (c. 4BC–AD65)

Our state of mind is never precisely the same. Every thought we have of a given fact is, strictly speaking, unique, and only bears a resemblance of kind with our other thoughts of the same fact . . . Experience is remolding us every moment, and our mental reaction on every given thing is really a resultant of our experience of the whole world up to that date.

William James (1842–1910)

For, what is the peculiar character of the modern world – the difference which chiefly distinguishes modern institutions, modern social ideas, modern life itself, from those of times long past? It is, that human beings are no longer born to their place in life, and chained down by an inexorable bond to the place they are born to, but are free to employ their faculties, and such favourable chances as offer, to achieve the lot which may appear to them most desirable.

John Stuart Mill (1806–1873)

It is remarkable how easily and insensibly we fall into a particular route, and make a beaten path for ourselves.

Henry David Thoreau (1817–62)

A tower of nine storeys begins with a heap of earth.
A journey of a thousand miles starts from beneath
your feet.

Lao Tsze (c.604–531BC)

Man cannot discover new oceans until he
has courage to lose sight of the shore.

Author unknown

A slavish bondage to parents cramps
every faculty of the mind.

Mary Wollstonecraft (1759–97)

In the mid-journey of our life below,
I found myself within a gloomy wood
No traces left the path direct to show.

Alighieri Dante (1265–1321)

Young men think old men are fools;
But old men know young men are fools.

George Chapman (1559–1634)

Art is long and time is fleeting,
And our hearts though stout and brave,
Still, like muffled drums are beating
Funeral marches to the grave.

Henry Wadsworth Longfellow (1807–82)

I remember, I remember,
The fir trees dark and high;
I used to think their slender tops
Were close against the sky;
It was a childish ignorance,
But now 'tis little joy
To know I'm farther off from heaven
Than when I was a boy.

Thomas Hood (1799–1845)

The best guide is not he who, when people are in the right path, merely praises it, but he who shows them the pitfalls and the precipices by which it is endangered . . .

John Stuart Mill (1806–73)

I wish I could remember the first day,
First hour, first moment of your meeting me,
If bright or dim the season, it might be
Summer or winter for aught I can say.
So unrecorded did it slip away.

Christina Rossetti (1830–94)

At thirty a man suspects himself a fool;
Knows it at forty, and reforms his plan;
At fifty chides his infamous delay,
Pushes his prudent purpose to resolve;
In all the magnanimity of thought
Resolves: and re-resolves; then dies the same.

Edward Young (1683–1765)

Like the winds of the sea are the ways of fate;
As the voyage along through life;
'Tis the will of the soul
That decides its goal,
And not the calm or the strife.

Ella Wheeler Wilcox (1855–1919)

All old men might have, and some old men really have, knowledge which it is altogether impossible that a young man, however great his capacity, should possess a very large measure of, namely, that which is derived from personal experience.

John Stuart Mill (1806–73)

A man among children will be long a child, a child among men will be soon a man.

Proverb

I delight in the idea of being a grandmama; to be that at thirty-nine and to look and feel young is great fun, only I wish I could go through it for you, dear, and save you all the annoyance. But that can't be helped. I think of my next birth being spent with my children and a grandchild. It will be a treat!

Queen Victoria (1819–1901)

Lovers grow cold, men learn to hate their wives,
And only parents' love can last our lives.

Robert Browning (1812–89)

There's night and day, brother, both sweet things; sun, moon and stars, brother, all sweet things; there's likewise a wind on the heath. Life is very sweet, brother; who would wish to die?

George Borrow (1803–81)

I do not weep from a sense of bereavement . . . but for the wreck of talent, the ruin of promise, the untimely dreary extinction of what might have been a burning and a shining light. My brother was a year my junior . . . Nothing remains of him but a memory of errors and sufferings.

Charlotte Brontë (1816–55)

I miss my mother till this moment when I am near as old as she was (sixty, 10th June 1888): I think instinctively still of asking her something, referring to her for information, and dream constantly of being a girl with her at home.

Caroline Oliphant (1766–1845)

What is the worst of woes that wait on age?
What stamps the wrinkle deeper on the brow?
To view each loved one blotted from life's page,
And be alone on earth, as I am now.

Lord Byron (1788–1824)

All the worlds a stage, and all the men and
    women merely players.
They have their exits and their entrances,
    and one man in his time plays many parts.

William Shakespeare (1564–1616)

As the clear light is upon the holy candlestick, so is
the beauty of the face in ripe age.

The Bible, Ecclesiasticus, 23:17

Childhood is scarcely more lovely than a cheerful, kindly, sunshiny old age.

Lydia Mary Child (1802–80)

For while a youth is lost in soaring thought
And while a mind grows sweet and beautiful,
And while a spring-tide coming lights the earth,
And while a child, and while a flower is born,
And while one wrong cries for redress and finds
A soul to answer, still the world is young.

Lewis Morris (1833–1907)

My heart leaps up when I behold
A rainbow in the sky:
So was it when my life began
So is it now I am a man:
So be it when I shall grow old,
Or let me die.

William Wordsworth (1770–1850)

The Soul . . . overcomes Birth, Death, Sorrow, and Age; and drinketh deep the undying wine of Amrit.

Bhagavad Gita, Book 14

We do not believe immortality because we have proved it, but we try for ever to prove it because we believe it.

James Martineau (1805–1900)

Youth beholds happiness gleaming in the prospect. Age looks back on the happiness of youth and, instead of hopes, seeks its enjoyment in the recollection of hope.

Samuel Taylor Coleridge (1772–1834)

A good leg will fall; a straight back will stoop; a black beard will turn white; a curled pate will grow bald; a fair face will wither; a full eye will wax hollow: but a good heart, Kate, is the sun and moon; or rather the sun and not the moon; for it shines bright and never changes, but keeps his course truly.

William Shakespeare (1564–1616)

The soul is born old but grows young. That is the comedy of life. The body is born young and grows old. That's life's tragedy.

Oscar Wilde (1854–1900)

Thy Lord hath decreed that ye worship none but Him, and that ye be kind to parents. Wether one or both of them attain old age in thy life, say not to them a word of contempt, nor repel them, but address them in terms of honour.

And out of kindness, lower to them the wing of humility, and say: 'My Lord! Bestow on them thy Mercy even as they cherished me in childhood.'

The Qu'ran 17:23–24

It is He Who brings out the living from the dead, and brings out the dead from the living, and Who gives life to the earth after it is dead: and thus shall ye be brought out (from the dead).

The Qu'ran 30:19

As he came forth of his mother's womb, naked shall he return to go as he came, and shall take nothing of his labour, which he may carry away in his hand.

The Bible, Ecclesiastes 5:15

That way, the highest way, goes he who shuts
The gates of all his senses, locks desire
Safe in his heart, centres the vital airs
Upon his parting thought, steadfastly set:
And, murmuring OM, the sacred syllable,
Emblem of Brahm – dies, meditating Me.

Bhagavad Gita, Book 8

When I am dead, my dearest,
Sing no sad songs for me;
Plant thou no roses at my head,
Nor shady cypress tree:
Be the green grass above me
With showers and dewdrops wet:
And if thou wilt, remember,
And if thou wilt, forget.

Christina Rossetti (1830–94)

Why fear death? It is the most beautiful
adventure in life.

Charles Frohman (1860–1915)

Mine be the breezy hill that skirts the
    down;
Where a green grassy turf is all I crave,
With here and there a violet bestrown,
Fast by a brook, or fountain's murmuring
    wave;
And many an evening sun shine sweetly
    on my grave.

James Beattie (1735–1803)

Man is a noble animal, splendid in ashes,
    and pompous in the grave.

Sir Thomas Browne (1605–82)

The evil that men do lives after them;
The good is oft interred with their bones.

William Shakespeare (1564–1616)

Here lie I, Martin Elginbrodde
Ha'e mercy o' my soul, Lord God,
As I wad do, were I Lord God
And ye were Martin Elginbrodde.

Author Unknown

You never know what life means till you die:
Even throughout life, tis death that makes life live,
Give it whatever the significance.

Robert Browning (1812–89)

The good mariner, when he draws near the port,
furls his sails, and enters it softly; so ought we to
lower the sails of our wordly operations, and turn
to God with all our heart and understanding.

Alighieri Dante (1265–1321)

They who make the least of death, consider it
as having a great resemblance to death.

Marcus Tullius Cicero (106–43BC)

Thus let me live, unseen, unknown;
Thus unlamented let me die;
Steal from the world, and not a stone
Tell where I lie.

Alexander Pope (1688–1744)

Remember, o friend, your end.

Now you are strong and fit, filled with ambition,
    boasting of your achievements, but all your
    success is a mere passing shadow.

Remember you are made of clay, and to clay you
    will return.

Now you are healthy and handsome, filled with
    energy, proud of your work; but all your joys
    are mere passing shadows.

Remember your life is the breath of God, which at
    death will depart.

Now your life on earth is solid and stable, but
    soon it will dissolve, your body crumbling to
    dust.

Remember, o friend, your end.

Author unknown

The *Great Eastern* or some of her successors will perhaps defy the roll of the Atlantic, and cross the seas without allowing their passengers to feel that they have left the firm land. The voyage from the cradle to the grave may come to be performed with similar facility. Progress and science may perhaps enable untold millions to live and die without a care, without a pang, without an anxiety . . . But it seems unlikely that they will have such a knowledge of the great ocean on which they sail, with its storms and wrecks, its currents and icebergs, its huge waves and might winds, as those who battled with it for years together in the little craft . . .

Fitz–James Stephen (*written in* 1862)

Finding Joy

O Son of God, change my heart.
Your spirit composes the songs of the birds
  and the buzz of the bees.
Your creation is a million wondrous miracles,
  beautiful to look upon.
I ask of you just one more miracle: beautify
  my soul.

Prayer (Author unknown)

Eternal love made me.

Alighieri Dante (1265–1321)

I make and unmake this Universe:
Than me there is no other Master, Prince!
All these hang on me
As hangs a row of pearls upon its string.
I am the fresh taste of the water; I
The silver of the moon, the gold o' the sun,
The word of worship in the Veds, the thrill
That passeth in the ether, and the strength
Of man's shed seed. I am the good sweet smell
Of the moistened earth, I am the fire's red
    light,
The vital air moving in all which moves.

Bhagavad Gita, Book 7

Few folk hae seen oftener than me Natur getting up i' the morning . . . Never see ye her hair in papers.

John Wilson (Christopher North) (1785–1854)

A violet, by a mossy stone
Half hidden from the eye!
Fair as a star, when only one
Is shining in the sky.

William Wordsworth (1770–1850)

I do not know what I may appear to the world, but to myself I seem to have been only like a boy playing on the seashore, and diverting myself in now and then finding a prettier shell or a smoother pebble than ordinary whilst the great ocean of truth lay all undiscovered about me.

Sir Isaac Newton (1642–1727)

To see a World in a Grain of Sand
And a Heaven in a Wild Flower
Hold Infinity in the palm of your hand
And Eternity in an hour.

William Blake (1757–1827)

Though we travel the world over to find the beautiful, we must carry it with us or we will find it not.

Ralph Waldo Emerson (1803–82)

There's music in the sighing of a reed;
There's music in the gushing of a rill;
There's music in all things, if man had ears;
The earth is but the music of the sphere.

Lord Byron (1788–1824)

I consider an human soul without education like marble in the quarry, which shows none of its inherent beauties till the skill of the polisher fetches out the colours, makes the surface shine, and discovers every ornamental cloud, spot, and vein that runs through the body of it.

Joseph Addison (1672–1719)

I have a hut in a wood; only my Lord knows it; an ash tree closes it on one side and a hazel like a great tree by a rath on the other.

The size of my hut, small, not too small, a homestead with familiar paths. From its gable a she-bird sings a sweet song in her thrush's cloak.

A tree of apples of great bounty like a mansion,
   stout; a pretty bush, thick as a fist, of small
   hazel nuts, branching and green.
Fair white birds come, herons, seagulls, the sea
   sings to them, no mournful music; brown
   grouse from the russet heather.
The sound of the wind against a branching wood,
   grey cloud, riverfalls, the cry of swan,
   delightful music!

Author unknown

The clear cuckoo sings to me, lovely discourse, in
   its grey cloak from the crest of the bushes;
Truly – may the Lord protect me! – well do I write
   under the forest wood.

Author unknown

Earth teach me stillness as the grasses are stilled
with light

Earth teach me suffering as old stones suffer with
memory

Earth teach me humility as blossoms are humble
with beginning

Earth teach me caring as the mother who secures
her young

Earth teach me courage as the tree which stands
all alone

Earth teach me limitation as the ant which crawls
on the ground

Earth teach me freedom as the eagle which soars
in the sky

Earth teach me resignation as the leaves which
die in the fall

Earth teach me to forget myself as melted snow
    forgets its life
Earth teach me to remember kindness as dry
    fields weep for rain.

Prayer (Author unknown)

You never enjoy the world aright till the sea itself
    floweth in your veins,
till you are clothed with the heavens and crowned
    with the stars,
and perceive yourself to be the sole heir of the
    whole world.

Thomas Traherne (*c.*1636–74)

To gild refined gold, to paint the lily,
To throw a perfume on the violet,
So smooth the ice, or add another hue
Unto the rainbow, or with taper-light
To seek the beauteous eye of heaven to garnish,
Is wasteful, and ridiculous excess.

William Shakespeare (1564–1616)

Loveliness needs not the foreign aid of
    ornament,
But is, when unadorn'd, adorn'd the most.

James Thomson (1700–48)

There is a pleasure in the pathless woods;
There is a rapture on the lonely shore,
There is society, where none intrudes,
By the deep sea, and music in its roar.

Lord Byron (1788–1824)

And still they gazed, and still the wonder grew,
That one small head should carry all he knew.

Oliver Goldsmith (1728–74)

. . . and the great sun
Looked with the eye of love through the golden
    vapors around him;
While arrayed in its robes of russet and scarlet
    and yellow
Bright the with sheen of the dew, each glittering
    tree of the forest
Flashed like the palm-tree the Persian adorned
    with mantles and jewels.

Henry Wadsworth Longfellow (1807–82)

The twilight hours like birds flew by,
As lightly and as free;
Ten thousand stars were in the sky,
Then ten thousand on the sea.
For every wave, with dimpled face,
That leaped upon the air,
Had caught a star in its embrace
And held it trembling there.

Amelia Welby (1819–52)

Moonlight is sculpture; sunlight is painting.

Nathaniel Hawthorne (1804–64)

Who can paint like Nature?
Can imagination boast amid its gay creation,
Hues like hers?

James Thomson (1700–48)

The mountains and the hills shall break forth before you into singing, and all the trees of the field shall clap their hands.

The Bible, Isaiah 1:12

The verie essence, and, as it were, springe-heade and orgine of all musicke, is the very pleasaunte sounde which the trees of the forest do make when they growe.

Author unknown

The streams with softest sound are flowing,
The grass you almost hear it growing,
You hear it now, if e'er you can.

William Wordsworth (1770–1850)

Look upon the rainbow, and praise him that made it; very beautiful it is in the brightness thereof; it compasseth the heaven about with a glorious circle, and the hands of the Most High have bended it.

The Bible, Ecclesiasticus, 13:11–12

Spring hangs her infant blossoms on the trees, Rock'd in the cradle of the western breeze.

William Cowper (1731–1800)

Who can hold a fire in his hand
By thinking on the frosty Caucasus?
Or cloy the hungry edge of appetite
By bare imagination of a feast?
Or wallow naked in December snow
By thinking on fantastic summer's heat?

William Shakespeare (1564–1616)

The roaring cataract, the snow-topt hill,
Inspiring awe, till breath itself stands still.

Robert Bloomfield (1766–1823)

A thing of beauty is a joy for ever;
Its loveliness increases; it will never
Pass into nothingness.

John Keats (1795–1821)

There is in souls a sympathy with sounds;
How soft the music of those village bells,
Falling at intervals upon the ear
In cadence sweet, now dying all away.

William Cowper (1731–1800)

What would the world be, once bereft
Of wet and of wildness? Let them be left,
O let them be left, wildness and wet;
Long live the weeds and the wilderness yet.

Gerard Manley Hopkins (1844–89)

There is no frigate like a book
To take us lands away
Nor any coursers like a page
Of prancing poetry –
This travel may the poorest take
Without offence of toll –
How frugal is the chariot
That bears the human soul.

Emily Dickinson (1830–86)

Life is like music; it must be composed by ear,
feeling and instinct, not by rule.

Samuel Butler (*c.*1612–80)

I went to the woods because I wished to live
deliberately, to front only the essential facts
of life, and see if I could not learn what it
had to teach, and not, when I came to die,
discover that I had not lived.

Henry David Thoreau (1817–62)

Poems are made by fools like me,
But only God can make a tree.

Joyce Kilmer (1886–1918)

If the devil doesn't exist, but man has created him, he has created him in his own image and likeness.

Feodor Dostoevsky (1821–81)

Know too, from Me
Shineth the gathered glory of the suns which
    lighten all the world:
From Me the moons draw silvery beams, and
    the fire fierce loveliness.
I penetrate the clay, and lend all shapes their
    living force:
I glide into the plant, root, leaf and bloom,
To make the woodlands green with springing
    sap

Bhagavad Gita, Book 15

Behold, thy Lord said to the angels: 'I am about
to create man from clay:
When I have fashioned him (in due proportion)
and breathed into him of My spirit, fall ye
down in obeisance unto him.'

The Qu'ran 38:71–72

No one ever talks about the beauty of Cairo, ever
gives you the least idea of this surpassing city. I
thought it was a place to buy stores at and pass
through on one's way to India, instead of its being
the rose of cities, the garden of the desert, the pearl
of Moorish architecture, the fairest, really the
fairest, place of earth below.

Florence Nightingale (1820–1910)

To my taste there is nothing so fascinating as spending a night out in an African forest, or plantation; but I beg you to note I do not advise anyone to follow the practice . . . It is like being shut up in a library whose books you cannot read, all the while tormented, terrified and bored. And if you do fall under its spell, it takes all the colour out of other kinds of living.

Mary Kingsley (1862–1900)

But you, my friend, must know that the true artist is as useful as the priest or warrior, and that when the artist respects the true and the good, he is on a road which God will bless without ceasing.

George Sand (1804–76)

My first act of free-will shall be to believe in free will . . . I will go a step further with my will, not only act with it, but believe as well; believe in my individual reality and creative power.

Williams James (1842–1910)

We are born with faculties and powers capable almost of anything, such, at least, as might carry us further than can easily be imagined; but it is only the exercise of those powers that gives us ability and skill in anything, and leads us towards perfection.

John Locke (1632–1704)

Each man has his fortune in his own hands, as the artist has a piece of rude matter, which he is to fashion into a certain shape.

Johann Wolfgang von Goethe (1749–1832)

Earth is here so kind, just tickle her with a hoe and she laughs with a harvest.

Douglas Jerrold (1803–57)

Emotion, not thought, is the sphere of music: and emotion quite as often precedes as follows thought.

Hugh Haweis (1838–1901)

Music is an invisible dance, as dancing
is a silent music.

Jean Paul (1763–1825)

It is vain to do with more what can be
done with fewer.

William Occam (*c.*1270–1349)

It is the greatest invention man has ever
made, this of marking down the unseen
thought that is in him by written characters.

Thomas Carlyle (1795–1881)

It is the treating of the common-place with the feeling of the sublime that gives to art its true power.

Jean François Millet (1814–75)

Music is the crystallisation of sound.

Henry David Thoreau (1817–62)

No productiveness of the highest kind, no remarkable discovery, no great thought which bears fruit and has results, is in the power of any one; such things are exalted above all earthly control. Man must consider them as an unexpected gift from above, as pure children of God, which he must receive and venerate with joyful thanks . . . as a vessel found worthy for the reception of such divine influence.

Johann Wolfgan von Goethe (1749–1832)

Dream delivers us to dream, and there is
no end to illusion.

Ralph Waldo Emerson (1803–82)

We heard a strange sound in the Bainriggs wood,
as we were floating on the water; it seemed in the
wood, but it must have been above it, for presently
we saw a raven very high above us. It called out,
and the dome of the sky seemed to echo the sound.
It called again and again as it flew onwards, and
the mountains gave back the sound, seeming as if
from their centre; a musical bell-like answering to
the bird's hoarse voice.

Dorothy Wordsworth (1771–1855)

Music is but wild sounds civilised
into time and tune.

Thomas Fuller (1608–61)

And why take ye thought for raiment?
Consider the lilies of the field, how they
grow: they toil not, neither do they spin:
And yet I say unto you, That even Solomon
in all his glory was not arrayed like one of
these.

The Bible, Jesus, Matthew 6:28–29

Cauliflower is nothing but cabbage
with a college education.

Mark Twain (1835–1910)

When in the world beauty is recognized to
be beautiful, straightway there is ugliness.

Lao Tsze (c.604–531BC)

The best part of beauty is that which
a picture cannot express.

Francis Bacon (1561–1626)

Sure there is music even in beauty, and the
silent note which Cupid strikes, far sweeter
than the sound of an instrument. For there is
music wherever there is harmony, order or
proportion.

Sir Thomas Browne (1605–82)

I was never weary of great churches. It is my favourite kind of mountain scenery. Mankind was never so happily inspired as when it made a cathedral.

Robert Louis Stevenson (1850–94)

There are not enough words in all Shakespeare to express the merest fraction of a man's experience in an hour.

Robert Louis Stevenson (1850–94)

He who resolves never to ransack any mind but his own will be soon reduced from mere barrenness to the poorest of all imitations: he will be obliged to imitate himself, and to repeat what he has before repeated.

Sir Joshua Reynolds (1723–92)

The true order of going is to use the beauties of earth as steps along which one mounts upwards for the sake of that other Beauty, going from one to two, and from two to all fair forms and from fair forms to fair actions, and from fair actions to fair notions, until from fair notions he arrives at the notion of absolute Beauty, and at last knows that the essence of Beauty is.'

Plato (427–347BC)

No one can make clear to another who has never had a certain feeling, in what the quality or worth of it consists. One must have musical ears to know the value of a symphony; one must have been in love one's self to understand a lover's state of mind. Lacking the heart or ear, we cannot interpret the musician or the lover justly.

William James (1842–1910)

Sobriety dimishes, discriminates, and says no; drunkenness expands, unites, and says yes. It is in fact the great exciter of the 'Yes' function in man. It brings its votary from the chill periphery of things to the radiant core . . . Not through mere perversity do men run after it. To the poor and the unlettered it stands in the place of symphony concerts and literature . . .

William James (1842–1910)

About 11, I home, it being a fine moonshine; and so my wife and Mercer came into the garden, and my business being done, we sang till about 12 at night with mighty pleasure to ourselfs and neighbours, by their casements opening.

Samuel Pepys (1633–1703)

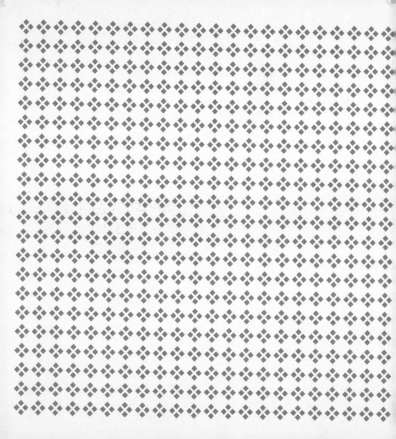